Praise for *Nursery of Heaven*

"I am sure that my Saint Mom and my holy Dad who suffered two miscarriages — my Dad even the loss of his most beloved Spouse and then of his daughter Mariolina at the tender age of six — are very united to the spouses who experience the great pain of loss. May my parents' heroic sufferings and full trust in Divine Providence, so well described in this very important book, be a source of consolation for them. I assure my prayers to my saintly parents so that, through their intercession, these spouses and parents may have peace, serenity and hope in their heart, and continue to trust completely in Our Lord and in His infinite Love for us."

— ***Gianna Emanuela Molla,***
Last daughter of Saint Gianna and Pietro Molla

"With faith, compassion, and raw honesty, this book speaks to the hearts and souls of grieving parents from all walks of life. The Scriptures, stories from the lives of the saints, and words of wisdom gained from painful personal experience all come together in a way that will help heal hearts and renew the faith of all those who grieve."

— ***Danielle Bean,***
Writer and speaker

"This book will help people understand the pain of pregnancy loss. It is helpful for those who have experienced loss to know they are not alone and helpful to those who love them in understanding this often hidden experience and how to help."

— ***Vicky Thorn,***
Foundress, Project Rachel

"For those who have suffered from infertility or still struggle with it, those who have lost a child in miscarriage at any stage, and those who have had a stillborn son or daughter, these personal accounts help us all come together to honor and celebrate faith, hope, love and everlasting life."

—Sheila Liaugminas,
Author, broadcaster, journalist, and, most importantly, mother

"How to pastorally accompany those who have lost a baby is one of those delicate situations that require the wisdom of experience. Miscarriage, stillbirth, and infant loss are painful experiences that require a sensitive pastoral approach. Some situations are so painful that the witness of those who have walked the same path is the only way forward. It is this insight that makes *Nursery of Heaven* a powerful resource for those struggling with the loss of a child. Over the years I have learned from listening to those who shared what was helpful and what was not. If a joy shared is twice the joy, then a sorrow shared is half the sorrow. *Nursery of Heaven* is a perfect companion for those who have lost a child and those who seek to accompany them."

—Fr. Luke Mary Fletcher, C.F.R.
Chaplain of the National Blue Army Shrine of Our Lady of Fatima

Cassie Everts and Patrick O'Hearn

Nursery of Heaven

Miscarriage, Stillbirth, and Infant Loss in the Lives of the Saints and Today's Parents

SOPHIA INSTITUTE PRESS
Manchester, New Hampshire

Cover by Mike Fontecchio, Faith & Family Publications

Cover image: *The Nursery of Heaven* by Michael Corsini

Sophia Institute Press
Box 5284, Manchester, NH 03108
1-800-888-9344
www.SophiaInstitute.com

Sophia Institute Press is a registered trademark of Sophia Institute.

paperback ISBN 979-8-88911-306-5

ebook ISBN 979-8-88911-307-2

Library of Congress Control Number: 2024939740

Second printing

This book is lovingly dedicated to Our Mother of Sorrows
and our little ones we have lost:

Elizabeth Atkinson
Adam Michael Atkinson
Dylan Marinus Ballard
Shay Angelica Ballard
Luke Michael Blanton
Sarah Ruth Blanton
Alex Bell
Ephesus Therese Bell
Jesse Bell
Sloane Sienna Bell
Ada Marie Day
Noel Regina Everts
Frances Everts
Simon Everts
Cecilia Everts
Gabriel Everts
Michael Fetsko
Angela Michelle Giganti
Xavier Paul Giganti
Blaise Mark Giganti
Peter McClone Jr.
Gerard McClone
Samuel Mary McIlroy
Thomas John O'Hearn
Angelica Rose O'Hearn
George Swannack
Isabel Lucia Tafoya

What I wish to say to the mothers who have lost children is this: we have been mothers; we have had this great gift. The amount of time does not matter: one month, two months, a few hours. What matters is that we have had this gift … and it is something that can never be forgotten.

— Servant of God Chiara Corbella Petrillo

Contents

PART III
PRACTICAL WISDOM

PART IV
REFLECTIONS, PRAYERS, AND SCRIPTURE PASSAGES

PART V
TOOLS FOR THE JOURNEY

Nursery of Heaven

Acknowledgments

We would like to thank our spouses for their unfailing support and for sharing in the mystery of Christ's suffering.

We would also like to thank our families and friends for their encouragement.

We thank our little ones in Heaven, whose prayers made this book possible. Forgive us for the times when we have forgotten you.

We would like to thank in a special way all the fathers and mothers who contributed their stories. Thank you for your vulnerability and for sharing the intimate story of your baby's life. We ask God to reward you with the greatest prize, which is to see His face and to see your little ones.

We would also like to thank Michael Corsini for our beautiful book cover. We commissioned Michael to paint the image, *The Nursery of Heaven*, after Patrick received an inspiration before the Blessed Sacrament. This painting depicts our departed children with the Blessed Mother in the Nursery of Heaven.

We would like to thank Sophia Institute Press for publishing this important work.

Finally and most importantly, we give thanks to God for the gift of our lives and for the Holy Spirit and Our Lady for inspiring this work.

We pray that *Nursery of Heaven* brings healing and hope to your grieving heart.

Introduction

Dear Reader,

You may find yourself picking up this book because in some way your life has been impacted by the loss of a baby through miscarriage, stillbirth, or in infancy. Perhaps, you are the mother, father, grandparent, aunt or uncle, or a close friend. I offer my deepest sympathy and condolences as you grieve the loss of a precious and sacred life. As you journey through the words in this book, may it be a balm to your soul, a consolation in your grief, and a threshold of hope in your suffering.

Miscarriage: A word that never entered my mind or made me pause for a second. A word I had heard spoken by my own mother and mother-in-law, who had mentioned their losses in passing, but one that still never penetrated my heart. In my naiveté, I thought that miscarriage was something that happened in past generations but had become uncommon in modern times, especially since I had never heard much about it.

Fast forward to my own miscarriage a year into my marriage, when the word took on a whole new meaning. The grief was tangible, and my heart was left raw. I could not stop thinking about what had happened, my pain never seemed to heal, and a feeling of loneliness set in.

Now, every time I hear the exciting news of someone expecting, my first thought and quiet prayer is, Please dear God, do not let them lose this child, protect this child they carry.

Miscarriage and stillbirth both describe pregnancy loss but refer to different times during a pregnancy. The Centers for Disease Control and Prevention (CDC) defines miscarriage as "loss of a baby before the twentieth week of pregnancy," while "a stillbirth is loss of a baby at twenty weeks of pregnancy and later."[1]

The American College of Obstetricians and Gynecologists (ACOG) reports that 10 percent of all pregnancies end in miscarriage, while other resources, such as the American Pregnancy Association, believe the rate may be as high as 25 percent. According to the CDC, "about 1 in 175 births" in the United States result in a stillbirth. This is also the same rate of infant loss — that is, babies who do not survive the first year of life.[2] Numbers aside, the loss of a baby is heart-wrenching and painful at any point in a pregnancy.

While I felt that I was alone, in reality I wasn't. All I had to do was look to my left and right while sitting in the pew on Sunday, and I would encounter many other couples who had experienced such a loss. Each of our stories is unique, our grieving handled differently and the path to healing distinct, but we are bound together by the loss we suffered. A quiet community in the Church exists, most not

1 Centers for Disease Control and Prevention, "Pregnancy and Infant Loss," last reviewed September 30, 2022, https://www.cdc.gov/ncbddd/stillbirth/features/pregnancy-infant-loss.html.

2 American College of Obstetricians and Gynecologists, "Early Pregnancy Loss," Practice Bulletin no. 200, November 2018, https://www.acog.org/womens-health/faqs/early-pregnancy-loss; American Pregnancy Association, "Symptoms and Signs of Miscarriage," https://americanpregnancy.org/getting-pregnant/pregnancy-loss/signs-of-miscarriage/; Centers for Disease Control and Prevention, "What Is Stillbirth?" last reviewed September 29, 2022, https://www.cdc.gov/ncbddd/stillbirth/facts.html.

saying anything, but their minds wandering to the small soul who is no longer with them, and their hearts left hurting.

Somewhere between my fourth and fifth miscarriages, my husband and I attended a beautiful prayer service for those who had experienced the loss of a baby. It was a simple service organized by a couple of parishioners, but incredibly moving. I was surprised by how many couples attended. At the end we were invited to come forward to receive a candle and say something about our babies if we chose to. Women of all ages came forward. An elderly lady in particular remains etched in my mind. She said she had never talked about her miscarriage, and fighting back her tears, she told us she had decided the night of the service to name her baby, who had been lost decades ago.

Although decades had passed, her baby was never forgotten. Each child lost leaves a footprint with us forever, much more than just a memory. The reality is a mother carries cells in her body from her miscarried or stillborn child for the rest of her life; this is known as microchimerism. So while we may think of our babies as departed, they are literally a part of us. They are much nearer to us than we could ever imagine. And these cells are also passed to future children, linking our living children with their siblings in Heaven.

I was thrilled when I heard this book was being written. I wish I had such a book when I struggled through my own losses. I am often asked by others who have a loved one who has experienced miscarriage, stillbirth, or infant loss for books to read, and I struggle to find something to suggest. There are not enough resources available, especially ones written from the beautiful perspective of the Catholic Faith.

While this book may be difficult to read at times, recalling our own pain and sorrow, I hope that it also brings encouragement from the stories of the saints as well as today's parents. Here are beautiful stories from the lives of the saints, ordinary people who carried the same crosses we each face today. Yet, in their sorrow they show us how to draw closer to Christ in our suffering. We hear also from modern-day couples, who like each of us were not prepared to journey through the heartache and the loss of our baby. Still, in their own struggles they offer much encouragement and hope.

I pray that the words in this book will bring consolation to your own grieving heart. That in the pain and immense suffering you are journeying through, you will know the God who loves you and has not abandoned you. I pray that in the sorrow of the cross you carry, you will one day experience the joy of the resurrection. Clinging to the promise of new life given to us by our Savior, may you never lose hope.

Whether the loss is recent or years ago, may we look forward to the day when, God willing, we will hold our precious little ones in our arms after they run to meet us saying, "Mommy is home, Mommy is finally home!"

With many prayers,
Cassie Everts

When my wife and I exchanged our vows, we envisioned having many children. After all, my wife was the third of thirteen children. We saw a large family as a blessing from God. I think many faith-filled married couples secretly believe God "owes" them children — as if children are a right rather than pure gift. After not getting pregnant after seven months of trying, we were somewhat discouraged. My wife received some chiropractic treatment, which helped her scoliosis, and we prayed a novena to St. Thérèse of Lisieux. Shortly after, we received the greatest news of our life — we were expecting. Thanks be to God, our first child, Jude Martin, was born nine months later. Following Jude's birth, though, we had the misfortune of having two miscarriages in a span of fourteen months.

When my cousin and his wife suffered a miscarriage with their first child, they lamented that the Church seems to care more about abortion than a miscarried child. There may be some truth to this, and both abortion and miscarriages need to be addressed with mercy and love. Many parents who have lost a child through abortion, miscarriage, stillbirth, or infant loss grieve in a similar way. Though the years pass, many never forget the day of their child's death or their due date.

Unfortunately, few parishes have a cemetery for preborn babies. Often, our pastors, relatives, and friends do not know what to say, so they say nothing. As a result, those who have had a miscarriage, stillbirth, or infant loss are left to grieve silently. Many in our parishes have no idea of our hidden sorrow, asking innocently, "Are these all your children? Isn't it time to add another one to the family?"

During a somewhat heated exchange with an atheist coworker over abortion, I told him that I knew what it was like to lose two children. After clarifying that I meant having miscarriages, he said something that pierced my heart. He asked, "Why didn't your God save them?" For a few moments, I was shrouded in darkness as my faith was put to the test. God then gave me the grace to respond, "Whether a child lives a few weeks or eighty years, their life has value." That night, I asked God in prayer why my children had died, and I felt His reply, "Patrick, I wanted your children more than you. After all, they are mine." God willing, I will understand this better in Heaven. For now, though, I must live with the mystery.

The Catholic Church offers hope for those whose children have died without the sacrament of Baptism. In 2007, Pope Benedict XVI approved the International Theological Commission's findings regarding "The Hope of Salvation for Infants Who Die without Being Baptized." One line stands out: "There are reasons to hope that God will save these infants precisely because it was not possible to do for them what would have been most desirable — to baptize them in the faith of the Church and incorporate them visibly into the Body of Christ."[3] Certainly, God sees parents' desire for Baptism for their deceased child. Baptism is necessary for salvation, but God can also give His grace apart from the sacraments, "for with God nothing will be impossible" (Luke 1:37).

For fathers and mothers who have lost a child, I pray this book brings some consolation and healing to your sorrows. You are not alone. Your relatives and fellow parishioners may never understand your suffering because they have never experienced the loss of a child. But those who have, do understand — and our Mother of Sorrows knows your pain better than anyone. When Our Lady experienced Jesus' Crucifixion, you were on her mind. Her heart was pierced just as yours is.

The Russian novelist Fyodor Dostoevsky is often credited with these striking words: "The darker the night, the brighter the stars, the deeper the grief, the closer is God!" God is so close to you, dear brother and sister of the Cross. He is lifting you up at this very moment to Calvary ... to rest your head on His pierced heart. He will never let go of you or your beloved child.

One of my friends, Sr. Bethany Madonna, S.V. (Sisters of Life), once wrote me a beautiful note after I told her of our miscarriage. She cited a line from a poem: "Look for me in the nursery of heaven." In fact, Colton Burpo, whose life is chronicled in *Heaven Is for Real,* said, "The women in heaven — especially Mary — are involved with raising the kids."[4] What a consoling thought: that the Blessed Mother

3 International Theological Commission, "The Hope of Salvation for Infants Who Die without Being Baptised," January 19, 2007, The Holy See, https://www.vatican.va/roman_curia/congregations/cfaith/cti_documents/rc_con_cfaith_doc_20070419_un-baptised-infants_en.html.

4 Mark Ellis, "Mary Oversees Nursery in Heaven, Burpos Say," God Reports, May 6, 2014, https://www.godreports.com/2014/05/mother-mary-oversees-nursery-in-heaven-burpos-say/.

watches over both our children in Heaven and those on earth. I pray that all of us, God willing, will be reunited with our little loved ones, who eagerly await us in the Nursery of Heaven, where we will one day hold them in our arms forever.

With many prayers,
Patrick O'Hearn

Part I

THE SAINTS

CHAPTER 1

The Saints and Child Loss (1300–1900)

Before we consider modern-day stories of child loss, we will examine the lives of the saints. After all, the saints are our greatest models of virtue. We must never forget that the saints experienced everything we do, both the good and the bad. So we are in the best company—though when it comes to child loss, no one wants to be in that number. In our suffering, we can often feel so alone, that our grief is unique. In fact, others have suffered far worse.

When we read about the lives of the saints, we do not see much about miscarriages, stillbirth, or child loss. But many of them must have suffered through miscarriages, stillbirths, or lost siblings, since most came from large families. A dear friend of mine said he was deeply affected by his mother's miscarriages. Everyone suffers when a child dies, from grandparents to siblings. Those who have lost a child should take some consolation that the suffering they experienced can turn them into a saint, as seen by the following examples.

St. Alphonsus Rodriguez and Maria Suarez

We rightly praise the saints for their lengthy fasts, fervent prayers, and works of mercy. Unfortunately, this can keep them on a pedestal, making them seem so unlike us and our lives. St. Alphonsus Rodriguez, though, had a lot in common with the average Catholic today. Born on July 25, 1532, in Spain, St. Alphonsus took over his father's wool business when he died unexpectedly. At twenty-six, he married Maria Suarez, and they had three children. Over the next five years, two of their children died, as did Maria. Alphonsus became a widower at the age of thirty-one. Perhaps the grief of losing her two young children contributed to Maria's early death.

In his sorrow, Alphonsus turned to a life of prayer and penance. Sadly, he would lose his third child a few years later. With no wife or children left, Alphonsus felt the stirrings of a religious vocation. At the age of forty, he left behind his prosperous business and entered the Jesuits. Because Alphonsus's childhood education was cut short as a result of his father's death and his own poor health, he was accepted under the condition that he would be a lay brother rather than a priest. As a humble doorkeeper, many laypeople, including government officials, sought his advice. He also assisted the poor whenever possible and imagined that each person who came to his door was God Himself. He was an inspiration to future saints such as St. Peter Claver, as well as the famed Jesuit poet Gerard Manley Hopkins.

Although there is no documented story, Br. Alphonsus likely counseled a young father or mother who had a miscarriage, stillbirth, or infant death. Perhaps he helped a young widower or widow. Although he was not a priest, Alphonsus's sympathy and support spoke volumes to the people from all walks of life whom he counseled. The greatest saints were the most compassionate, because they experienced the most suffering, sometimes the same as the very people they were counseling. An old priest once told me he never realized how painful miscarriages were until he counseled a few mothers. Our hearts long for shepherds and friends like St. Alphonsus, who enter our pain by their support and sympathy rather than maintaining silence. St. Alphonsus Rodriguez's feast day is October 30.

St. Catherine of Sweden and St. Catherine of Siena

As the fourth child of St. Bridget of Sweden, St. Catherine's life closely paralleled her mother's. Both were widowed at a young age, and both later entered religious life, living lives of asceticism, piety, and charity to the poor. St. Catherine spent her final years as the superior of a convent founded by her mother. Yet, a key difference in their lives is that St. Bridget gave birth to eight children while St. Catherine gave birth to none. The latter decision was made from love rather than being due to selfishness or infertility. Specifically, St. Catherine and her husband took a perpetual vow of chastity, living as brother and sister in Christ. Yet St. Catherine of Sweden is the patron saint against miscarriages. Ironically, she and St. Catherine of Siena are forever linked, not only by their names, but as intercessors against miscarriages — even though neither had any children.

So why does the Church entrust these two fourteenth-century saints with such a noble mission before the throne of God? Their lives offer some clues into their role as patrons against miscarriages. St. Catherine of Sweden knew the longing to have a child. Coming from a large family, the call to motherhood was surely stamped in her soul. Yet God called her to be a spiritual mother to thousands rather than the biological mother of a few. Her beautiful and holy desire to have her own children was renounced for the sake of the Kingdom. In a mysterious way, St. Catherine of Sweden shared in the sufferings of many couples who are infertile or cannot bring a healthy child to birth. She willingly offered this sacrifice to draw nearer to God and to unite herself more fully with those who are unable to have children, as well as those who have lost children from miscarriage, stillbirth, or infant loss. As a wife and later as a sister, St. Catherine of

Sweden would likely have met some infertile couples and have offered her counsel and prayers.

St. Catherine of Siena's calling to intercede for couples with infertility issues is more personal. When St. Catherine of Siena's mother, Lapa, was forty years old, she gave birth prematurely to Catherine and her twin sister, Giovanna, who were her twenty-third and twenty-fourth children. Sadly, Giovanna did not survive. We do not know whether she was stillborn, had a genetic defect, or died due to complications from a premature birth. Tragically, St. Catherine of Siena's mother had buried half of her children as a result of the bubonic plague. In a mysterious way, Giovanna became Catherine's special intercessor in Heaven. Throughout her life, St. Catherine may have felt the lack of Giovanna's presence. They were sisters in the womb, created by God within moments of each other, but they had different destinies in life. One was to become a great saint and live thirty-three years as a Third Order Dominican nun; the other would become a saint and gaze upon the face of God immediately. Like St. Alphonsus Rodriguez and St. Catherine of Sweden, St. Catherine of Siena surely would have come to the aid of several mothers who had lost children at various stages of life. Witnessing her own mother's sorrow and tears over the loss of her siblings would have opened St. Catherine of Siena's heart to a life of compassion for those parents who bear the great cross of losing a child.

Both St. Catherine of Sweden and St. Catherine of Siena came from large families, yet they willingly renounced the desire for children to belong completely to God. Less apparent in their offering was their desire to be closer to humanity, which ultimately led them to identify more fully with couples who grapple with infertility. It has been said that priests choose to be alone so that others are not alone. The same thing applies to religious sisters, who renounce biological motherhood to be spiritual mothers to many. While on earth, the two Catherines accompanied their brothers and sisters in their sufferings, and continue to do so now in Heaven through their powerful intercession for parents who invoke their name for protection against miscarriage. It is appropriate that the saints we invoke for specific causes were once affected by the same crosses while on earth. St. Catherine of Sweden's feast day is March 24, while St. Catherine of Siena's is April 29.

Bl. Frédéric and Amélie Ozanam

"We are here on this earth to accomplish the will of Providence,"[5] wrote Bl. Frédéric Ozanam. The will of Providence can take many twists and turns, as seen in the lives of the saints.

Born on April 23, 1813, in Milan, Italy, Bl. Frédéric Ozanam and his family would soon return to their native France. One of fourteen children, Frédéric came face-to-face with death at an early age. Only three of his siblings would live to adulthood.

Homeschooled until the age of nine, Frédéric went through a "crisis of doubt" concerning his Catholic Faith in his teenage years, when an atheist classmate challenged his beliefs.

At the age of twenty, he founded the Society of St. Vincent de Paul to help the poor. The sight of the impoverished from the 1832 cholera epidemic moved young Frédéric to pity for his fellow brothers and sisters.

He later obtained a doctorate in law and letters. He would become a professor, renowned for his letters on law, literature, history, and social doctrine. He had a particular love for the Catholic author Dante Alighieri. And, despite his worldly success, Frédéric never forgot the poor families of Paris.

Besides his love for the poor, Frédéric fell in love with Amélie Soulacroix. At the age of twenty-eight, he married his bride on

[5] "Quotes Frédéric Ozanam," Vincentian Formation Network, https://vincentians.com/en/quotes-collection/frederic-ozanam-quotes/.

June 23, 1841. It was said that on the twenty-third of each month he would bring Amélie flowers to celebrate their anniversary day. Suffering would soon touch this young couple as Amélie experienced several miscarriages.[6] One article suggested that Amélie's first two pregnancies ended in miscarriage.[7]

As Amélie recovered at her parents' home, Frederic would write to her almost daily. We can only wonder what sentiments of love and consolation were shared between these two grieving hearts.

The couple would have a double rainbow (a baby after two miscarriages) when God blessed them with their daughter, Marie, in July 1845. Following this miracle, it was said that Frédéric "became less anxious and withdrawn and more open."[8]

Although their first four years of marriage were filled with infertility and loss, Providence was guiding this couple as they sought to abandon themselves to the will of God.

The couple was blessed with twelve years of marriage before Providence called Frédéric home at the age of forty, dying from tuberculosis. Frédéric and his two children would now be waiting and interceding for Amélie and Marie.

Bl. Frédéric once said, "Great men are those who never have the plan of their Christian destiny in advance, but they have let themselves be led by God's hand."[9] Bl. Frédéric's feast day is September 9.

[6] Amin de Tarrazi and Fr. Ronald Ramson, eds., *Ozanam: Husband and Father, Champion of Truth and Justice, Lover of the Poor, Founder of the Society of St. Vincent de Paul* (Strasbourg, France: Éditions du Signe, 1997), 18.

[7] Meg Hunter-Kilmer, "Saints Who Lost Children to Miscarriage," Aleteia, September 26, 2020, https://aleteia.org/2020/09/26/saints-who-lost-a-child-to-miscarriage/.

[8] De Tarrazi and Ramson, *Ozanam*, 18.

[9] "The Beatification of Frédéric Ozanam," The Holy See, https://www.vatican.va/jubilee_2000/magazine/documents/ju_mag_01091997_p-16_en.html.

Bl. Catalina de María Rodríguez and Manuel Antonio de Zavalía

On November 27, 1823, Bl. Catalina was born in Argentina. Her baptismal name was Saturnina Rodríguez. After praying the Spiritual Exercises of St. Ignatius of Loyola, seventeen-year-old Saturnina desired to become a nun. However, her spiritual director, Fr. Tiburcio López, told her to get married to his friend Manuel. Manuel, a recently widowed husband of two children, was unstable. Manuel told Saturnina that he would kill himself if she would not marry him. Fr. López insisted that Saturnina was now responsible for Manuel's soul.[10] As a result, Saturnina believed God was calling her to marriage.

Throughout Saturnina and Manuel's thirteen years of marriage, they experienced the cross of infertility. Saturnina took on a mother's heart as a stepmother to Manuel's children. But still, the couple desired to have children together.

Tragedy struck when Saturnina and Manuel's only child was stillborn. They named their daughter Catalina. At the age of forty-two, Saturnina lost her husband and decided to enter religious life. When she made her final vows, she took the name Sr. Catalina de María in honor of her deceased daughter.

After seven years of difficulties, Sr. Catalina founded a religious order of nuns called the Slaves of the Heart of Jesus, through which she would aid vulnerable women.[11] She would now be known as Mother Catalina de María. And it seems highly plausible that God allowed Mother Catalina's past sufferings, particularly her infertility and child loss, as a preparation for her new vocation to serve the most vulnerable women.

10 "This Argentine Nun's Cause for Beatification Is Advancing," Catholic News Agency, January 25, 2017, https://www.catholicnewsagency.com/news/35294/this-argentine-nuns-cause-for-beatification-is-advancing.

11 Ibid.

St. Louis and St. Zélie Martin

All five of St. Louis and St. Zélie's daughters became religious sisters, one of whom is St. Thérèse of Lisieux. What a testimony to this godly couple's virtue! But Louis and Zélie also buried four children over a four-year period, which caused them tremendous suffering. Their losses began with their first son, Marie-Joseph-Louis (Joseph), who died at the age of five months from erysipelas and enteritis. Their sixth child, Marie-Joseph-Jean-Baptiste, passed away at eight months from enteritis and bronchitis. Then, their fourth child, Marie-Helene, died from unknown causes at the age of five. Finally, the Martins said goodbye to their eighth child, Marie Melanie-Therese, when she was only seven weeks old. Zélie could no longer nurse at this point, and Melanie's wet nurse was an alcoholic and neglected her. After Melanie died in St. Zélie's arms, she penned these words: "Tell me that we didn't have misfortune! Finally, it is over, there is nothing else we can do. The best thing to do is to resign myself. My child is happy and that consoles me."[12]

The reality that Melanie's death could have been prevented only increased their pain. Because of this tragedy, Zélie refused to walk on the street where Melanie died. Like St. Zélie, many parents blame themselves when their child dies from an accident, a tragic event, or even a miscarriage.

St. Zélie would weep at the cemetery while visiting the graves of her two little boys. To add to her suffering, a friend told Zélie at Melanie's wake, only eight months after Helene's death, that "God surely sees that you could never cope with raising so many children, and he took four of them to Paradise."[13] Far from comforting St. Zélie, these words were extremely hurtful. Many of us have heard

12 St. Zélie Martin and St. Louis Martin, *A Call to a Deeper Love*, ed. Frances Renda, trans. Ann Connors Hess (Staten Island, NY: St. Paul's, 2011), 73.

13 Ibid., 82.

similar painful things from well-meaning family or friends, such as, "You can always have another one." These words miss the point, because we wanted *this* child, not another child in the future. It is not easy to move on when you have not yet grieved over the one who has been lost.

Losing a child affects both parents, fathers as much as mothers — though a father may grieve differently. Although there is little documentation concerning Louis's reaction to losing his children, he must have been devastated, as he was a few years later when his wife was diagnosed with the cancer that eventually took her life. He was described as "inconsolable." Clearly, St. Louis and St. Zélie were canonized because they kept their eyes fixed on the Cross and the hope of eternal life, even in the midst of their profound sufferings.

Because of their own tragedies, St. Louis and St. Zélie were keenly aware and sensitive to those around them. Suffering drew them out of themselves. A day after receiving a letter from her brother detailing the misfortune of losing his child and only son, Paul, who was stillborn, Zélie immediately expressed her compassion and sorrow. To her brother and sister-in-law, St. Zélie wrote,

> The tragedy you've just suffered saddens me deeply. You are truly being tested. This is one of your first sorrows, my poor sister! May God grant you resignation to his holy will. Your dear little baby is at his side. He sees you, he loves you, and you will see him again one day. That is a great consolation I have felt and still feel.
>
> When I closed the eyes of my dear little children and when I buried them, I felt great pain, but it was always with resignation. I didn't regret the sorrows and the problems that I had endured for them. Several people said to me, "It would be much better never to have had them." I

> can't bear that kind of talk. I don't think the sorrows and problems could be weighed against the eternal happiness of my children. So they weren't lost forever. Life is short and full of misery. We will see them again in heaven.[14]

The greatest sorrow many parents will experience in this life is losing a child, which can shatter one's faith. Rather than turn their backs on God, St. Louis's and St. Zélie's faith in God led them to believe that they would one day be reunited with their little ones again in Heaven. They never forgot about their deceased children. In fact, when their daughter Helene was suffering from an earache, St. Zélie felt inspired to seek the prayers of her son Joseph, who had died five weeks earlier. She told Helene to ask for her brother's intercession, and she was healed the following day. St. Louis and St. Zélie Martin's feast day is July 12.

[14] Ibid., 90–91.

CHAPTER 2

The Saints and Child Loss (1900–Present)

St. Josemaría Escrivá

St. Josemaría Escrivá experienced the loss of many siblings. In 1910, his youngest sister, Maria Del Rosario, died at nine months. Two years later another sister, Maria de los Dolores, died at the age of five, and one year later Maria Asuncion died at the age of eight. As a result, St. Josemaría told his mother, "Next year it's my turn." In response, Maria Dolores calmly declared, "Don't worry, I offered you to our Lady, and she will take care of you."[15] Maria's confidence in Our Lady proved to be well founded, as she not only took care of her son but helped guide him to be a faithful son of the Church. We must never forget that Our Lady is the greatest of mothers as she watches and defends us, especially at the hour of death! St. Josemaría Escrivá's feast day is June 26.

St. Gianna and Pietro Molla

Near the end of the second month of her last pregnancy, St. Gianna Beretta Molla was diagnosed with a huge fibromyoma (a benign

[15] Andrés Vázquez de Prada, *The Founder of Opus Dei: The Life of St. Josemaría Escrivá*, vol. 1, *The Early Years* (New York: Scepter, 2001), 52.

tumor) in her uterus. She was free to choose and decide among three different solutions:

> to have a hysterectomy (the safest solution for her life), to remove the fibromyoma with a surgery and put an end to that pregnancy with an abortion, to remove only the tumor and continue with the pregnancy. (This last was the riskiest solution for her life. The risk was this: the surgery necessary to remove the fibromyoma would have left a scar that could rupture during the pregnancy, causing a rupture to the uterus as well, with mortal risk for her and for the baby.) She chose the latter, and her daughter, Gianna Emanuela, was born by C-section because the natural childbirth did not work.[16]

Following the birth of her daughter, St. Gianna suffered septic peritonitis, a complication of delivery, and died seven days after giving birth. After her third pregnancy, according to the testimony of her brother, Dr. Ferdinando, who was taking care of her, Gianna had two miscarriages whose cause was never discovered.[17]

"My Mom and my Dad accepted these sufferings, but it was not easy," Gianna Emanuela said. "Throughout their lives, they always accepted God's Holy will, even when it was very difficult to accept, even when it was not immediately understandable. They always recognized that God's plan was the best plan. Despite their sorrows, they always completely trusted in Divine Providence."[18]

[16] Patrick O'Hearn, *Courtship of the Saints: How the Saints Met Their Spouses* (Gastonia, NC: TAN Books, 2023), 149.

[17] *The Journey of Our Love: The Letters of Saint Gianna Beretta and Pietro Molla*, ed. Elio Guerriero (Boston: Pauline Books and Media, 2014), 22.

[18] Gianna Emanuela Molla, *Witness of Gianna Emanuela Molla* to Patrick O'Hearn, March 8, 2024. Given as correspondence with the author.

In fact, those couples who prize human life more than their careers or their very selves find a miscarriage one of the greatest sufferings in this life. A few days before she died, St. Gianna told her husband, "Pietro, I have already seen the other side, and if you only knew what I saw. One day I will tell you. But because we were too happy, we were too well off with our marvelous children, full of health and grace, with all the blessings of heaven, heaven sent me back here to suffer some more, because it is not right to appear before the Lord without many sufferings."[19] St. Gianna may have seen their two miscarried babies along with other relatives during her glimpses of Heaven.

On April 28, 1962, St. Gianna died at the age of thirty-nine. Her daughter Gianna Emanuela related,

> She wanted to receive Holy Communion, at least on her lips, also on Thursday and Friday, when she was no longer able to swallow the Holy Particle. On April 28, 1962, Saturday in Albis, at dawn, she was taken back to her family home in Ponte Nuovo, as she wished and had asked of my Papa previously. She died in her nuptial bed, where she gave birth to my siblings, at 8 a.m.[20]

Less than two years later, Pietro said goodbye to his second child, Maria Zita (Mariolina), who died on February 12, 1964, at the age of six. He was alone to suffer this other huge sorrow, since his most beloved spouse was already in Heaven. When asked how he responded to the pain of losing his wife and daughter, he declared, "I clung to Jesus crucified, to the certainty that Gianna lived with God

[19] Giuliana Pelucchi, *St. Gianna, Her Life of Joy and Heroic Sacrifice* (Boston: Pauline Books and Media, 2019), 202.

[20] O'Hearn, *Courtship of the Saints*, 164.

in Paradise.... I relived this mystery of pain in an equally dramatic way when my daughter Mariolina died. Why does it happen?" Searching for answers to this mystery, especially when it seems as if God had "not accepted my supplications," Pietro came to the conclusion that "pain remains a mystery even in the light of our faith, and I have experienced in myself that the only way to accept it is that of Jesus crucified."[21] The pain of losing a child or wife never goes away, for every person is unique and unrepeatable. Either we cling to Christ Crucified or we numb our pain with fleeting pleasures. St. Gianna Molla's feast day is April 28.

Servants of God Cyprien and Daphrose Rugumba

When a couple prepares for the sacrament of Matrimony, God often hides their future crosses from them, unlike Christ who saw every suffering from the womb. Make no mistake, "Marriage is the cross and the cross is marriage."[22]

Before marrying Daphrose, Cyprien experienced the heartache of losing his fiancée Xaverina, who was likely murdered in the ethnic cleansings in Rwanda. In 1965, two years after Xaverina's tragic death, Cyprien wanted to honor Xaverina by marrying her cousin, Daphrose.

Their marriage began on rocky ground. The couple soon separated for eight months. "The reason for the separation was disturbing: Cyprien's family believed that Daphrose dabbled in the occult, and therefore, they advised him to disown his wife. Cyprien's family came to this unfounded conclusion when the couple's second child was born healthy, after the death of their first child from a miscarriage."[23] Sadly, some parents will blame themselves for

[21] Pietro Molla and Elio Guerriero, *Saint Gianna Molla: Wife, Mother, Doctor,* trans. James G. Colbert (San Francisco: Ignatius Press, 2004), 88–90.

[22] O'Hearn, *Courtship of the Saints,* 67.

[23] Ibid, 146–147.

their child's death, even with a miscarriage, stillbirth, or infant loss. Or, as in Daphrose's case, sometimes others falsely blame the mother for her child's death.

The couple would get back together after Cyprien acknowledged his error. And they would be blessed with ten children. More heartache ensued, however, when Cyprien fathered a child with another woman. But Daphrose's greatest sorrow was not Cyprien's infidelity, but his professed atheism.

Daphrose kept praying for her husband's conversion and steered her children in the Faith. She would take their children to Mass every week (including Cyprien's illegitimate daughter, whom Daphrose loved).[24]

Seventeen years later, Cyprien returned to the Faith after a near fatal illness in 1982. Daphrose's perseverance in prayer made all the difference. The couple's faith and marriage became stronger than ever. But the cross was looming in the distance.

Racial violence reached its peak in 1994 as a civil war broke out between the Hutus and the Tutsis. On April 7, 1994, after praying the entire night in their home's eucharistic chapel, Cyprien and Daphrose were murdered alongside six of their children.

According to author Caitrin Bennett, "When the attackers arrived, Daphrose begged for the chance to pray one last time in front of the Blessed Sacrament. A soldier struck her with the butt of his rifle, breaking her collarbone. The soldiers also shot at the tabernacle and stomped on the consecrated Eucharistic Hosts inside."[25]

At last, Cyprien and Daphrose and their six children would be reunited with their miscarried child and sibling in Heaven and receive from Christ a crown of martyrdom!

24 Caitrin Bennett, *Holier Matrimony: Rediscover the Church's Gifts to Married People* (Stockbridge, MA: Marian Press, 2024).

25 Ibid.

Servant of God Chiara Corbella and Enrico Petrillo

Although not yet canonized, Chiara Corbella Petrillo is on the path to sainthood. Her story is one of the most heartbreaking, but at the same time one of the most courageous and comforting, for anyone who has lost a child. Her life parallels that of St. Gianna Molla. In fact, she has been referred to as the "second Gianna." Born on January 9, 1984, Chiara lived a heroic life. A month after her wedding in October 2008, she and her husband, Enrico, conceived. What should have been the greatest news became the most heart-wrenching, as the ultrasound revealed that their daughter had anencephaly, which is the absence of a key part of the brain, skull, and scalp. Children with this condition usually live only a few hours or days after birth. On hearing this devastating news, "Chiara wept in the arms of her mother." Meanwhile, her husband was having dental surgery at the hospital. Not knowing how he would respond, an anguished Chiara begged Our Lady's help. She wrote, "From being condemned to a destiny without hope, I became filled with joy in seeing how the Lord saw this suffering."[26]

Advised to have an abortion, Chiara and Enrico refused due to their strong religious convictions. In Enrico's words, "She is our daughter. We shall accompany her as far as we can." In the meantime, some fellow Catholics caused them great suffering by telling them they were bad parents or even cursed. Moreover, some people would ask the gender of the baby when Chiara was pregnant. After saying it was a girl, a few would respond that the most important thing is that the baby is healthy. On one occasion, the usually serene Chiara became upset and declared, "Why? What if she is not?" Sadly, Maria died thirty minutes after her birth on June 10, 2009. The priest who

[26] Simone Troisi and Christiana Paccini, *Chiara Corbella Petrillo: A Witness to Joy*, trans. Charlotte J. Fasi (Manchester, NH: Sophia Institute Press, 2015), 28–29.

married them, Father Vito, baptized her. These parents heroically accompanied their child to the very end, and then the angels took her to Heaven. A funeral Mass was held on June 12, but only a few people attended. Why? "Most had declined to come because they did not know what to say," according to their friends.[27]

Reflecting on her choice of life over death, Chiara once beautifully declared:

> If I had aborted her, I do not think that I would have remembered the day of the abortion as a day of celebration, a day in which I had been liberated of something. It would have been a moment that I would have tried to forget, a moment of great suffering. But the day of Maria's birth I shall always recall as one of the most beautiful days of my life, and I shall tell all my children that the Lord wishes to send us that they have a special sister who is praying for them in heaven.[28]

A few months after losing Maria, Chiara became pregnant again. People regularly said to them that this child will be a "great joy," as if "Maria was a child we must forget," said Enrico. Unfortunately, an ultrasound showed that their child was missing one leg and part of an arm. When they heard this news, they asked God, "Where are you taking us?"[29] Another ultrasound revealed that their child had no kidneys, which meant that it would also die shortly after birth. Enrico and Chiara once again refused an abortion, against their doctors' wishes. Their son, Davide, was born on June 24, 2010, and baptized immediately. He lived for thirty-eight minutes. His funeral Mass was celebrated two

[27] Ibid., 32, 36, 44–45.

[28] Ibid., 43.

[29] Ibid., 55–56.

days later. Sadly, fewer people attended Davide's funeral than Maria's, just as Our Lord had fewer friends the closer he neared Calvary.

A few months after losing Davide, Chiara became pregnant a third time. This time their child had no birth defects. To their shock, however, during her fifth month of pregnancy, the doctors found a cancerous lesion on Chiara's tongue. Though she underwent a surgical procedure, she insisted that her baby's life be spared at all costs. After her child's birth on May 30, 2011, Chiara had another surgery. Unfortunately, over the next year, the cancer metastasized to a breast, her liver, lungs, and an eye. Chiara died on June 13, 2012, while wearing her wedding dress. She went to be with her two children in Heaven at the age of twenty-eight, having been married only three years.

On their son Francesco's first birthday, Enrico and Chiara wrote him a letter. Chiara would die a few weeks later. They wrote, in part,

> Dearest Frankie,
>
> Whatever you do will have sense only if you see it in terms of eternal life.
>
> If you truly love, you shall be aware of it by knowing that nothing truly belongs to you because everything is a gift.
>
> We loved your brother and sister, Maria and Davide, and we have loved you, knowing that you were not ours; that you were not for us. And so it must be with everything in life. Everything that you have does not belong to you; that is so you can make it bear fruit.
>
> Do not ever be discouraged, my son. God does not ever take anything away from you. If he takes something from you, it is only because he wishes to give you so much more.

> Thanks to Maria and Davide, we are more in love than ever with eternal life, and we have stopped being afraid of death. Therefore, God has taken from us in order to give us a bigger heart and to be opened to receiving eternity during this [earthly] life.[30]

Their words ought to fill the hearts of every father and mother who has lost a child. The saints knew that everything is a gift, especially children. When these saints lost their children, they knew it was not forever. And as a result, their focus turned toward Heaven. As Our Lord reminds us, "For where your treasure is, there will your heart be also" (Matt. 6:21). Besides Our Lord Himself, these parents' greatest treasure on earth was their children, so it was only natural for them to fall even more in love with Heaven, where God and their babies await them. While there were days and even years of intense agony and sorrow over their lost children, they allowed their faith to be the compass guiding them daily to the thought of seeing God face-to-face, along with their babies running toward them at their entrance into Heaven.

No one is immune to suffering. If there is one thing for certain, Calvary is not some distant memory of the past; it is relived in our lives daily. But so too is the Resurrection. The saints and the following contemporary stories reveal that death is the most painful event any of us will experience in our short lives, but through the Resurrection, we have hope that all will be well one day — perhaps not in this life, but for sure in Heaven. Life goes on, which is often easier for those around us who have never experienced such a profound tragedy. For those of us who have lost a child, we might never fully move on, for a part of us is lost, but we must never lose hope, because Jesus has conquered sin and death — and holds out the hope of eternal life.

[30] Ibid., 160.

There is no simple remedy to take away the pain of losing a child. No book or wise counsel can immediately end our agony. Yet reading about how God has helped other couples through similar trials offers hope that we are never alone in our sufferings. May the following modern-day stories give you some consolation in your current sufferings and inspire you to fall more in love with eternal life, where, God willing, we will be reunited with our little ones.

Part II

Today's Parents

CHAPTER 3

MISCARRIAGE

God, Where Are You?

Cassie Everts

IT WAS THE MOST wonderful time of the year, Christmas, and I could not wait for my husband, Aaron, and me to make the six-hour drive home to spend it with my family. Earlier in the month, we had celebrated our one-year wedding anniversary, and we felt like newlyweds on top of the world, as I was just a few days shy of twelve weeks pregnant.

The month before, we had seen my family and told them we were expecting. We still exchanged Christmas gifts with my siblings, so I handcrafted a Christmas list and included baby items to break the news. I can still feel the excitement when what we were telling them clicked and their faces reacted to the surprise — especially my mom, who was elated!

We arrived in Minnesota a few days before Christmas, so we could see my extended family of aunts, uncles, and cousins. On December 22, my mom took Aaron, me, and my younger brother out to dinner and to do some last-minute shopping. With my birthday just a few days after Christmas, she treated me and bought some maternity clothes as a birthday gift. I wasn't showing yet, but I was looking forward to the day when a bump would appear and I would be able to fit into maternity clothes.

My sister-in-law had just lent me her copy of *What to Expect When You're Expecting*. I started reading it that night. Around 2:00 a.m., I woke up with a stomachache and went to the bathroom. I lay in bed thinking I must have eaten something that didn't agree with me or perhaps I was coming down with a bug. I fell back asleep, but soon woke up again. This time, the ache was more like a cramp. I mentioned this to my husband and began looking through the book, searching for "miscarriage." I did not actually think that was what was happening, though.

I tossed and turned as I tried to ignore what I was feeling, but I couldn't fall back to sleep. I lay awake, focusing on the pain and beginning to pray that my intuition was wrong. The cramps soon turned into sharp pain, making it difficult to walk or move. Then I noticed some spotting.

I made my way to my mom, who was sleeping on the couch since she had given us my parents' room. I told her what was happening, and we made plans to see a doctor in the morning. By 5:00 a.m., the spotting had turned to bleeding, and I then knew. The next two hours were a blur as my blood loss increased. As we waited for the clinic to open, I never left the bathroom. Around 7:00 a.m., I passed out. Aaron and my dad quickly got me into the car as my mom called the ER to make sure a doctor was present, since it was a small-town hospital.

I remember lying in the sterile emergency room as the doctor searched for a heartbeat with a doppler device. I was begging God for a miracle, still clinging to a thread of hope. I recalled stories through history of children being made well, babies being brought back to life. Still, no heartbeat was found.

The doctor ordered an ultrasound, which required a twenty-minute drive to the next town. When we weren't praying together, I sat quietly, continuing to beg God for a miracle. Since I was still weak and lightheaded, they put me in a wheelchair. My mind was a blur.

We had to drive back to the ER for the doctor to give us the results. We made our way there and waited. As soon as he entered the room, I could tell from his expression that the news wasn't good. Aaron stood by my side, holding my hand. "I am sorry to tell you that your baby has passed and is no longer with you." The tears instantly streamed down my face. As I looked up, Aaron was wiping his eyes and my parents were fighting back tears.

My gut had told me that this would be the news, but my heart had been in denial. The hope I had held onto was ripped away. It was the day before Christmas Eve. Couldn't the Christ Child have saved my baby? I vaguely heard the doctor explain something about my progesterone level being extremely low for how far along I was. It didn't mean anything to me, and I really didn't care about it then. I just wanted him to find a heartbeat.

We drove back to my parents' house, and I just wanted to be left alone. Aaron sat with me on the bed and held me as we both cried. His words didn't offer me any comfort. I was numb. How could God have allowed this to happen? Why didn't He save my baby? Why didn't He hear my prayers? I had no answers to my questions.

It was Christmastime, but my joy had vanished. All I had to do was think about what happened for just a moment and the tears and sobs would begin again. I sat through Christmas Mass feeling more alone than ever, with everyone around me rejoicing, singing hymns of glad tidings and joy. I could barely get myself to mouth the words without starting to cry again. So many references to a baby being born triggered my emotions, which were still so raw.

It is our family's tradition to open gifts after Christmas dinner. I dreaded the thought of unwrapping the presents to find baby items for which I no longer had a baby. How would I react? Unknown to me, my younger brother, who was nineteen at the time, took it upon himself to drive an hour each way to the closest shopping mall on the busiest shopping day to buy me all new gifts.

A few days after the miscarriage, we named our baby Noel Regina: Noel, since it was so close to Christmas; and Regina, after Aaron's aunt, who is a religious sister and whose birthday it was the day our baby passed.

Once back home, I had a follow-up appointment with my ob-gyn and had some blood work done to make sure my hormone levels had gone back to normal. The doctor seemed sympathetic about what had happened, but her tune changed when I asked whether miscarriage is something to be concerned about. Her reply was, "Miscarriage is common, something natural that happens. We don't worry about it or show concern until you have had at least three or maybe even four." Three or four? Was she serious? I couldn't imagine having to go through this three or four more times before a doctor would try to discover what could be causing it to happen.

I decided to take the rest of the time between Christmas and New Year's off to have time to recover, both physically and emotionally. I did a lot of praying and journaling, but the longing for my child was still present. The doctor's office called with the test results. Today, I can still hear the voice on the other end: "I wanted to let you know that all of the product from conception is taken care of. Is there anything else I can help you with?" I couldn't believe what I heard. *Product?* She was using medically sterile terms with no hint of empathy. This was my baby, not a product. A *baby*—loved, longed for, and greatly missed.

I continued to grieve, sometimes wondering if my heart would ever find healing. I noticed, however, that as my husband continued to comfort me, his grief seemed to have dissipated. As the weeks went on, I continued to mourn and tried to understand why this happened. I began to grow frustrated, as it seemed he had already gotten over the loss. Why did he no longer appear sad? Didn't he love this baby? How could he just get over it? Doesn't he understand what happened?

Needless to say, arguments ensued as we tried to understand each other's feelings. No one had told me how hard a miscarriage would be on my marriage. More than ever, I felt so alone; not even my husband understood. What I didn't realize was that he was grieving, too; he was just processing the loss in his own way.

My husband's grief was seeing me suffer, not being able to take away my pain or lift me out of my sadness, no matter how hard he tried. His frustration came in wanting things to go back to normal. He wanted our marriage to return to how it was before the loss. More than ever, he wanted his wife back, complete with her joy.

As much as the pain never really left, I wanted to conceive again but was terrified to do so. It was recommended that we wait a few months before doing so. In the meantime, I called to inquire about the words I heard mumbled in the ER about progesterone. The doctor who saw me when I miscarried had encouraged me to look into getting my hormone levels checked. Even though it was only my first miscarriage, he thought it was worth looking into.

I didn't want to risk having another miscarriage and experiencing all the heartache, pain, and grief again without first making sure nothing was medically wrong. One of my sisters-in-law recommended a doctor who was a family practitioner, not an ob-gyn, but who was trained in NaProTechnology and monitoring hormones throughout pregnancy. She was able to squeeze me into her schedule.

I left my initial appointment with my head spinning, feeling more frustrated than when I had walked in. There was so much information to process, let alone discerning what tests we wanted to pursue and how much we were willing to spend. After all, maybe my first miscarriage was just a fluke rather than an indication that it would recur. We decided to proceed with the ultrasounds and blood tests to monitor my hormones during different parts of my cycle.

A year passed, and it was Christmas again. We traveled to my parents as we always did. I worried how I would feel, a year later in the same place. Could I handle my emotions, or would I find myself faking my joy once again at Christmas Mass?

I had ordered a floral arrangement in honor and remembrance of our little Noel to have as a centerpiece at Christmas dinner. On December 23, my mom presented me with a beautiful Christmas ornament adorned with the word *Noel* for us to hang on our tree.

Getting ready for Christmas Eve Mass the next day, I was startled when I heard the sound of a baby. I didn't think anyone was upstairs, but I thought perhaps my nephews had stopped over without me knowing. I walked out of the bathroom expecting to see them, but there was no one. The sound was clear in my ears, not a figment of my imagination. Some people may think it was just in my mind, but I know what I heard. It was a soft little coo, the voice of a small child that I can still distinctly hear to this day.

The small voice was a gift, the greatest gift I received that Christmas. As we prepared to celebrate God's greatest gift to mankind, the Infant Jesus, God was reaching down from Heaven that night and allowing me to feel the love of my little babe.

After months of waiting, I was finally at peace about being pregnant again. Thirteen months after losing our first baby, I felt that my heart had reached a level of healing that would allow me to make it vulnerable a second time, despite knowing the risk in doing so.

Following the NaPro protocol, we did everything according to the book: Clomid, progesterone, human chronic gonadotropin (HCG), and more progesterone. I was excited and filled with so much hope. My family happened to be visiting us on the day of my seven-week ultrasound. While I hadn't told friends or coworkers, I had decided to tell my parents and siblings about the pregnancy. As we sat together at breakfast, my father led us in a beautiful prayer, asking God for there to be life and health for the baby I carried, and for Aaron and me to be protected from miscarriage and loss.

I was confident that everything was going to be fine, and I was looking forward to sharing the first ultrasound pictures with my family upon returning from the appointment. All throughout the ultrasound I kept wondering why they never showed me any pictures or pointed out a heartbeat, so I finally asked. The technician responded that if there was something to show me, she would. My heart sank. I knew what the news was going to be. As much as my heart wanted to once again deny the reality, I knew the fate of my baby.

We returned to the hotel where my family was staying, and I said nothing. I acted as if there were no ultrasound that morning. I forced myself to smile and laugh as I played with my toddler nephews, distracting myself from reality. Finally, someone broke the ice, asking how everything went. Exchanging a quick glance with Aaron, I knew I had to tell them. They had showed me nothing; there were no pictures, no heartbeat that I was able to listen to. I tried to be strong, acting as if it didn't really bother me.

A few hours later, my doctor called to go over the ultrasound results with me. She said, "I'm afraid to tell you we could not detect a heartbeat. Perhaps it is still too early to tell." I knew the thread of hope she was giving me was a single, thin thread, almost invisible. With Aaron standing next to me, I hung up the phone, and there were no words we needed to exchange as I fell into his arms and sobbed. We said goodbye to our baby, Frances, on March 9, 2010, on the feast of St. Frances of Rome.

Again the feeling of loneliness overwhelmed me, but I received two cards of condolence after losing Frances that meant the world to me. I still have them today. They offered simple words of support, comfort, and love.

They say it is better to have loved and lost than never loved at all, but I now questioned whether this was true. The emptiness and hurt that again clenched my heart, the anger and loneliness that fell upon me, left me wishing I had never conceived. I wouldn't then be grieving over the loss of my baby and feeling this pain. I wouldn't have to go through the next several months acting like everything was okay, as if nothing ever happened, when the truth was that I was not okay.

Looking back, I now realize that, while I would not have had the pain and heartache of losing my child, I would have missed out on much. I would have never experienced the excitement that comes from seeing the two pink lines. The joy that you instantly wake up with knowing you are pregnant another day. The bond and hope only a mother knows. I would never have known the depth of love that is felt so immensely for the child in your womb.

On Mother's Day, we took my mother-in-law out for dinner along with Aaron's brothers and their wives. At the end of dinner one of Aaron's sisters-in-law stood up with a beautiful vase of flowers and handed them to me. She said, "I can't imagine how hard Mother's Day is for you and the pain you feel, the longing for children. We want you to know that you are a mother to all of our children and every day we are praying for you and Aaron, that God will bless you with children." I will never forget how much that meant to me, as Mother's Day was always a day that seemed only to be a reminder of what I didn't have.

We continued to follow NaPro protocol and seek our doctor's advice. She strongly suggested that we travel to Omaha to have exploratory surgery with Dr. Thomas Hilgers at the Pope Paul VI Institute. Over the course of two months, we went to Omaha twice for appointments, tests, and two surgeries. As I lay on the operating table about to be put under, Dr. Hilgers asked if he could place a rosary blessed by

Pope Benedict XVI in my hand. An incredible peace came over me, and my first beautiful memory of coming out of surgery was feeling the beads of the rosary in the palm of my hand.

In 2011, I was certain we would conceive and have a successful pregnancy. We had done everything we could to treat infertility and to address the issues that could have been causing the miscarriages. When I found out I was pregnant for the third time, I was filled with incredible hope that this would be it; this time I would finally be able to hold my baby.

I attended a college reunion with some of my close friends, and seeing so many of them pregnant or holding a baby, I decided to announce that I too was expecting, even though I was only five weeks at most. I so longed to be a part of that group, awaiting the arrival of my baby and finally caressing one in my arms.

When I returned home, I had a routine blood test to check my levels, only to receive a call from my doctor later that day saying that they hadn't increased as much as they should have. We would repeat the blood work and go from there. I knew what the numbers had to be in order for the baby to be alive, and I wasn't there.

I repeated the blood work and was able to see the numbers before any phone call was received; they had not increased. I stared blankly at the computer, at numbers that told the fate of my baby. Anger overcame me as I cried out to God. Why didn't You save my baby? We did everything we were supposed to. We have been faithful; we have prayed every novena, gone on pilgrimages, made sacrifices, and all for naught. God, where are You? Why are You not hearing me? Why have You abandoned me?

Holy Week was right around the corner, and we would soon be entering the Holy Triduum. I was unable to get my mind to focus on Jesus' Passion. I could only think about one thing — my third baby I was having to say goodbye to. How could I prepare for the joy of Easter when every day felt like Good Friday?

Since it was Holy Week, we named our little one Simon. We prayed, "We give our sweet Simon back to You, Jesus. May he help You carry Your Cross, may he alleviate Your pain and bring healing to Your wounds."

I couldn't seem to hold back the tears during the Easter Vigil. In addition to having already started bleeding earlier in the day, the homily seemed to pierce my heart. The priest kept mentioning the hope of Easter. After every Good Friday, we have the joy of Easter. I bit my lip and squeezed my husband's hand to try to prevent myself from completely breaking down and sobbing during Mass. I longed to feel the joy of Easter, to feel the hope, to feel the presence of God. I felt like my life was stuck at Good Friday and constantly repeating. For years now, Lord, we have been praying and suffering as our hearts so desperately long for the gift of a child. When will we feel the joy, when will we experience Easter Sunday and see life brought to barren ground?

Now three of our babies were with the Lord, my faith shaken, and our marriage struggling. There had to be answers, more that could be done. Perhaps more hormone injections or another surgery. Something, anything. I remember browsing the computer and looking at maternity clothes or walking through the baby aisles at the store, still imagining that someday there would be a baby.

I will never forget the phone call I received that July. We were vacationing at Lake Koronis in central Minnesota, and Dr. Hilgers called me personally to discuss my most recent miscarriage and lab work. He spoke words that I will never forget. "I am sorry," he said. "There is nothing more we can do for you. We have tried everything." I bit my lip so hard it hurt, trying to numb the pain and fighting back the tears until I got off the phone with him.

Aaron was sitting on the bed next to me and heard everything. He held me tightly as I hung up the phone and I collapsed in his arms, sobbing uncontrollably. My hope gone, the dream of carrying a baby in my womb and holding one in my arms now taken away. Like Hannah in the Bible, "She was deeply distressed and prayed to the LORD, and wept bitterly" (1 Sam. 1:10). The last threads I clung to were ripped from my grasp, along with what seemed like every fiber of my heart. Having to grapple with the reality of the words the doctor spoke was incredibly painful. To come face-to-face with having to finally let go of the longing to see my belly grow, feel my baby kick, and when nine months were complete, to caress him or her in my arms.

I began to wonder if Aaron could still love me. I let questions arise in my mind that the Evil One was using to drive me further into despair. I wondered if Aaron would have married me if he had known that I might never be able to carry a child for him. Would he have stood at the altar and said, "I do," if he could have seen the future and what it held?

Still, we continued to bind our marriage together in prayer. We continued to pray novena after novena. We committed ourselves to praying the fifty-four-day Rosary novena continuously, turning to Our Lady for her intercession — a mother who had suffered immensely yet still knew joy. Her heart was pierced, seeing her own Son suffer and die, yet she was faithful to the end.

Through prayer and waiting, I slowly set my own will aside to accept God's will. I began praying less for a baby and more for God's perfect will to be done in our lives, in our marriage and family. I let go of the dream of being able to give birth to a baby and focused on what God's dream was for me. Little by little, I began to feel peace.

Through it all, both Aaron and I felt God placing the call of adoption on our hearts. Our Lady heard our prayers and made it known through multiple signs and affirmations. It became very evident that adopting was not something we were seeking, but was truly God's will for us. So we did our research and signed on with an agency for a domestic adoption, only to find out a month later that I was pregnant again, which meant the agency dropped us. I was so confused. We were so certain adoption was God's will, yet here I was finding myself pregnant again and the door seemed to be closing.

In the midst of the confusion, I was still excited and hopeful seeing those all-too-familiar pink lines show up again. With this pregnancy things were different. Every morning I would thank God for the child in my womb and pray in thanksgiving for the gift of one more day to have with my baby. On June 5, 2012, we said goodbye to our sweet Cecilia. "The Lord gave, and the Lord has taken away; blessed be the name of the Lord" (Job 1:21) were words I kept repeating in my mind and heart.

The passing of our little one came just days before traveling to Minnesota for my grandfather's funeral. While I was grieving both losses, I remember the isolation when I told my family about the baby I had just lost. I realize that their grief at my grandfather's passing occupied them, but it was almost as if I had had so many miscarriages that when I mentioned one more it didn't seem to matter — just another number.

Aaron and I continued to pursue adoption. Our Lady led us to the African country of Ghana. We had just received the referral pictures of our sons when I started having abnormal spotting that continued for two weeks. Realizing that this was more than just my period, I did a quick WebMD search for some possible reasons and learned that ectopic pregnancy could be the cause. During my lunch break, I bought a pregnancy test, thinking that I should at least rule that out before calling my doctor. To my surprise, the test was positive.

After work, I saw the doctor on call, and he confirmed I was indeed pregnant but was miscarrying. The next day, Aaron and I took off work to do some Christmas shopping and enjoy time together leading up to our anniversary weekend. While we were out, I received a call from my primary doctor. He had looked over the results and told me that I was experiencing an ectopic pregnancy. On our fifth wedding anniversary, December 1, 2012, we lost our angelic Gabriel.

I had never imagined that Aaron and I would still be trying to build a family after five years of marriage. Yet I also never expected we would be called so clearly to adopt. When we were standing at the altar, we thought we had it all figured out. We would wait six months or so after our wedding to get settled, buy our first house, and start our family. We expected that I would become pregnant within the first year or two, and I would be a stay-at-home mom. God had other plans. I wished I could go back to my twenty-three-year-old self and say, "Be ready, hang on, trust, and allow God to fulfill your dreams."

In a way, I think it is a grace that we do not know the road that lies ahead. It was a blessing that God did not give us a screenshot of the future, asking us to take one step at a time with Him. As with every couple, we said, "I do," not knowing what the future would hold, but trusting and knowing *who* held the future.

No matter how many times you experience a miscarriage, I discovered, it does not get easier. You may feel like you can navigate the waters better and know what you need to do as you go through the process. But each time is a profound loss, because every life is unique, precious, and beautiful, not just another statistic.

After so many years of clinging and grasping at my wants, I finally let God write his story. God placed adoption on our hearts, and we brought home our sons two and a half years later. A year later, I gave birth to our daughter, and twenty months after that I gave birth to our son. We had gone from zero to four children in a matter of two years.

Not all stories are like ours, but even in the wait, God is always present and working in our life. When nothing more than pain and the desire to be a mother consumes us, God has a plan. In our grief, God is molding our hearts. Though it often feels like He is using a chisel, we are being made new. When it seems as if God has abandoned us and we are alone, it is then that He is holding us so closely, pressing a kiss upon our forehead, saying, "My daughter, I am here. My love for you will never end."

CHAPTER 4

MISCARRIAGE

Live on Forever in Our Hearts

Patrick O'Hearn

I CAN STILL SEE it to this day—and will for the rest of my life. As I entered our house following work on that glorious May 2017 day, our little nineteen-month-old son, Jude, hid behind my wife to surprise me. And as he peeked out with my wife's prompting, he held a little sign that my wife made: "I'm going to be a big brother." I was in shock. It was one of the greatest moments of my life. A few hours later, I sent my brothers a text asking them to listen to the song "100 Years" by Five for Fighting because there was a secret message in the lyrics, and I wanted them to see if they could decode it. Within a few hours, I received a text: "Are you guys pregnant?" To which I responded: "YES!" Specifically, the lyrics read:

I'm thirty-three for a moment.
Still the man, but you see I'm a "they"
A kid on the way, babe
A family on my mind

I was thirty-three years old, my "Jesus year." My wife and I were so thrilled to welcome another child and a sibling to our little son, Jude.

Most couples wait until after fourteen weeks, around the start of their second trimester, to tell their family and friends they are pregnant, for fear of a miscarriage. But we told our family and close friends the great news right away and asked for prayers. I was so happy that the next day I offered my Mass intention for our baby's safety and in thanksgiving to God!

I don't know why, we asked everyone we told for their prayers. Something was different with this pregnancy. Each night, I would trace the Sign of the Cross with holy water on my wife's belly. I secretly longed for another son to be buddies with Jude and pictured him with my black hair. Jude has his mother's complexion, with sandy blond hair.

All was going well until Thursday, June 22. As I was taking a walk with Jude, Amanda's sister Esther, who was visiting us, ran to me in tears and said, "Amanda is bleeding." My mind went to the worst-case scenario: the baby is gone. I immediately sprinted into the house to find my wife in tears. "What does this mean?" I asked. It was June 22, the feast of St. Thomas More, a sixteenth-century English martyr who stood up to King Henry VIII on many things, one of which was his seeking a divorce. I immediately grabbed a second-class relic of St. Thérèse (a piece of her casket) and a third-class relic of Bl. Solanus Casey and placed them on Amanda's womb as I began to invoke these saints along with St. Thomas More. We were not about to surrender our child to the Lord. I texted a friend of mine who lived next to a Perpetual Adoration chapel, asking him to please stop in and pray for us. I also texted our family and a few other friends to implore God's mercy, if it be His will, to spare our child's life!

Amanda continued to bleed the following day, which was a Friday. We contemplated what to do, and decided we would see if the local pregnancy center could do an ultrasound on Saturday to give us peace of mind. (Ironically, this pregnancy center sits roughly one hundred yards from an abortion clinic.) To our surprise, a Mass was being celebrated at the pregnancy center, and it happened to be the feast of the Nativity of St. John the Baptist. I felt the Lord speak to us through the readings, particularly the first reading from Jeremiah, "Before I formed you in the womb I knew you, and before you were born I consecrated you" (1:5).

Later, during the Consecration, all I could think was, "Lord, please save these babies who are about to be aborted, but also save my child." Following Mass, there was Eucharistic Adoration. We were taken to a small room for a consultation. As we were waiting, we ran into a Catholic man who had just been praying at the abortion clinic, and he said that two babies had been saved. I shared with him that my wife was bleeding and we were not sure if she had a miscarriage but were seeking a miracle to keep our child alive. He assured me, "Your child will be fine. This will be the third miracle today." (The other two miracles were the two mothers who chose life.)

The director of the clinic asked that my wife have the ultrasound alone, as this was the protocol. In the meantime, I implored our Eucharistic Lord and Our Lady to spare my son! How ironic that a short distance away, some mothers were taking their children, who were the same age as our preborn child, to be killed, and here we are, begging God to save our child's life! I shed more tears. While in the chapel, another sidewalk counselor placed his arm on my left shoulder as I knelt in prayer. I never said anything to him about our baby, but he sensed that something was wrong.

On Sunday morning, just prior to leaving for Mass, my wife called me to the bathroom to show me the large clots of tissue she had lost. She and I embraced each other as we wept over our child, whom we so longed for. It seemed so unreal. During the homily, the priest spoke about St. Thomas More's martyrdom. Two things struck me during his homily: I was so grateful that our child had received through my wife's reception of Holy Communion, Viaticum, "bread for the journey," when he was living. Second, though this is my opinion, I believe my child was a martyr like St. Thomas More. In a mysterious way, I believe my child was pouring out his blood, united with Our Lord's on the Cross, to help save two babies at the abortion clinic. These insights came to me during Mass.

Upon leaving Mass, we told Amanda's sister that we were certain she had experienced a miscarriage, and more tears flowed. I told my wife I wanted to name our son Thomas John after St. Thomas More and St. John the Baptist. When we returned home, I offered to make pancakes. As I put on a random Pandora station on my iPhone, these lyrics played: "I'm fifteen for a moment. Caught in between ten and twenty." "God bumps" began to tingle down my arms. As I looked at my phone, it dawned on me that this was the song I had sent to my brothers the day we found out we were pregnant! I had not even "put a thumbs up" to save this song; it just "coincidentally" played, as people would say. But I believe God and my departed son were the DJs of that song, to remind me they are always near.

I immediately picked up Jude in my arms and began to circle him around in a dance as the sunlight shone on our kitchen floor. In that moment, I felt embraced by God's presence. I felt like our son Thomas John was smiling upon us. I consider that the third miracle: that our son, though dead, was fully alive now. God clearly wanted me never to forget that suffering does not have the last dance!

Later that day, I pushed Jude on his Radio Flyer bike, which also has a spot where someone can stand behind the cycle seat. Naturally, Jude was standing as I pushed him. In front of Jude was an empty seat as the air moved the pedals. In that instant, I pictured Thomas pedaling. My heart was still torn. At the same time, I thanked God for my beautiful son, Jude, and for all His blessings. Through this trial, I realized even more how sacred each life is.

On June 28, our anniversary, my wife took another pregnancy test, which revealed that there was still a significant level of HCG. The doctor at the pregnancy center told her to come in to see what was going on. This second ultrasound confirmed that my wife had miscarried.

While sadness and sorrow overwhelmed us, we had to slowly resign ourselves to God's will. Later that night, my wife gave me a gift—the movie *Heaven Is for Real.* I had read the book in one day a few years earlier, and the one thing that struck me the most was when the little boy met his miscarried older sister in Heaven. His parents had never told him about his older sister. In fact, she had no name, because his parents never named her. The young boy told his parents she looked like their mother. I had mentioned this movie before to my wife, because that incident left a profound impression on me. As we watched it that night, I longed to see our son even more someday.

Providentially, a day after our son died, my wife had a dream of a little boy with big ears, who looked like Jude. Was this Thomas? I would like to think so. Though it was too early to tell the gender, my wife jokingly said, "What if we get to Heaven and Thomas is a girl? Should we name her Thomasina?" I responded, "Well, she can be Agnes, as she would have been born shortly after her feast day." I still believe he was a boy!

On June 29, the feasts of St. Peter and St. Paul, exactly a week after my wife started bleeding, we had our son buried at St. Joseph's, a small cemetery for the Holy Innocents in Raleigh, North Carolina. The priest who baptized Jude graciously conducted the ceremony, which consisted of a few prayers and a sprinkling of holy water on our son's remains, which were enclosed in a four-by-four-inch wooden box with a picture of two angels on it. On this picturesque eighty-degree summer night, surrounded by pine trees, a few dear friends, and a giant statue of St. Raphael, I placed my son's little box in a small hole. I kissed the box one last time and then was asked to shovel dirt over his little casket. Tears continued to pour down my face. I never thought I would bury one of my children. I then placed a little gray, unmarked stone over the spot. I took Jude one last time and said, "Jude, this is where your little brother, Thomas, is buried."

Meanwhile, my wife's eyes were filled with tears, reminiscent of Our Lady of Sorrows, who held her son's battered and lifeless body in her arms. During our heartbrokenness, Jude started to smile at me — a way to remind us that all would be well. How beautiful that the Catholic Church does cherish and remember our miscarried babies, though some parishes and priests are more clearly devoted to the cause.

The day after Thomas's burial, I ran into the director of the pregnancy center and thanked her for helping us the previous Saturday. She knew that my wife had miscarried. She told me that five babies had been saved that Saturday, and two women had accepted Our Lord. I got "God bumps" again. I believe that my wife and son's suffering, joined with the Holy Sacrifice of the Mass, bore fruit.

On July 1, the Thirteenth Sunday of Ordinary Time, we attended the Saturday vigil Mass. The first reading, from 2 Kings chapter 4, spoke directly to Amanda and me as if God had chosen this reading precisely for us at this moment, particularly the words from the prophet Elisha.

> Later Elisha asked, "Can something be done for her?"
> His servant Gehazi answered, "Yes!
> She has no son, and her husband is getting on in years."
> Elisha said, "Call her."
> When the woman had been called and stood at the door,
> Elisha promised, "This time next year you will be fondling a baby son." (14–16, NAB)

A few hours after Mass, I asked Amanda what she thought of the readings, and she said that the last line from the first reading really jumped out at her. Although this turned out not to be the case (fondling a baby son in a year), God seemed to be calling us to more patience and trust. During our sufferings, God worked small miracles, like a song, the smile of our son, and the support of family and friends.

The days and months following our miscarriage did not get easier, as most of our friends began getting pregnant. Many of them never knew our hidden sorrows, since my wife did not want to tell them when they were pregnant. Furthermore, the stress from my wife's miscarriage literally made her sick. When our son's due date was approaching in mid-February, I tried to think of some tangible way I could remember Thomas John. And so I composed the following poem:

A Poem to My Son

We long to meet you someday!
Your life was like a shooting star.
You passed away too soon and now you live afar.
We think about you each and every day.

You would have been born this week.
Sadly, the world will never know you.
For you were gone like the morning dew.
We dream of you and your tiny feet.

We were so thrilled when you were conceived.
It was early May and our life would never be the same.
We could not wait to see your face and call you by name.
That day never came and still we must believe.

We longed to introduce you to your older brother.
He would have been your best friend.

Instead we are left wondering when our pain will end.
Send us another sibling we pray, Blessed Mother.

Still, no future child will ever replace you.
You were unique and unrepeatable.
So full of life and capable.
We longed for your debut.

It seems so unfair that you are no longer here.
Many around us have never known our pain.
You were clearly Heaven's gain.
In our hearts is where you are most dear.

Until you lose a child you will never know.
Move on, they say, time will heal.
God, please help us, as we kneel.
There is only one choice — surrender and follow.

Until we meet again, Thomas.
Know that we will never forget you.
In Heaven's nursery you have the best view.
Save us a spot when death draws near,
and we have our boarding pass.

May God keep you in His arms, dear son.
We pray Heaven is lots of fun.

Love,
Dad

In July 2018, I heard "100 Years Ago" for the first time since Thomas's death. I thought to myself, "Thomas is looking after us, good things are around the corner." I prayed a novena to St. Louis and St. Zélie Martin leading up to their feast day on July 12. I prayed for a baby and my wife's healing. She had high thyroid levels. A few weeks later, before our bone broth fast for a gut healing protocol, I asked my wife to take a pregnancy test as a precautionary measure. And to our great surprise and delight, we were pregnant. My wife couldn't believe it. My prayers had been answered.

We called the doctor right away, and immediately my wife was put on some natural pig hormones for her thyroid. We told our relatives to pray. My wife and I were happy but also cautious. We knew how her last pregnancy ended. I also called over a priest to give us a special pregnancy blessing, which assigns a guardian angel to this pregnancy. Things were looking good. I began to pray a Memorare every day for our baby's safety, entrusting this child to the Blessed Mother.

Amanda had an ultrasound and even heard the baby's heartbeat, something we weren't fortunate enough to do for Thomas, because we wanted to wait longer to get an ultrasound. Unfortunately, I was at work. My wife would return a week later for a follow-up appointment, because our baby's heart rate was lower than normal. Again, we summoned the family to pray.

My wife called to deliver the news I feared most. With anguish in her voice, she said "Patrick, there is no heartbeat, and the baby stopped growing at six weeks according to the ultrasound." I left my office to walk outside as tears rolled down my cheeks. We had tried for over a year, and this is what happened. We were beyond devastated. Only a few weeks earlier, we told our almost three-year-old son, "Jude, Mommy has a baby in her tummy." Jude asked about the baby the weekend after my wife's appointment. With tears in our eyes, we told him his sibling died. He didn't understand, but he needed to hear the truth. A part of me was not giving up, or at least perhaps I didn't want to come face-to-face with reality. I heard a story about a father whose child was stillborn. He immediately called every family member and friend he knew and asked for a miracle through the intercession of Ven. Fulton Sheen. The baby came back to life.

During First Saturday Mass, I felt inspired to seek Bl. Solanus Casey's intercession. I had a third-class relic of his, which I placed on the spot where he was born, in Oak Grove, Wisconsin, only an hour away from my wife's childhood home. I was praying for a miracle just like I did with Thomas, but it never came. After two weeks passed, I still kept praying for divine intervention, but my wife kept telling me that the baby was gone. Three weeks after the follow-up ultrasound, my wife started bleeding. That night, I held my sobbing wife in bed. In a mysterious way, it was like a martyrdom of both my wife and child, as a part of my wife died, too, along with her baby. Her dreams of holding this baby vanished in an instant, as did mine. She tried to collect most of the tissue so we could bury our child. We named her Angelica Rose since she would have been born near April 20, the birthday of Mother Angelica, the founder of the Eternal Word Television Network (EWTN).

While picking up groceries on the day we found out Angelica had no heartbeat, I saw the most beautiful little blond-haired girl, with the sun glowing over her head as she walked by me with her mother. She looked like my wife as a young girl. This was another sign from God. A week later, while I was working out, the song "I Love You Always Forever" by Donna Lewis randomly played on Pandora. I had not heard this song since my wife and I had danced to it on my birthday more than five years earlier, before we were married. As I listened to the lyrics, I paused for a second and felt it was Angelica who was singing to me. "I love you always forever. Near or far, closer together. Everywhere I will be with you."

A few days before my son's third birthday, we had our daughter buried immediately in front of her older brother, Thomas. As I laid our little girl in the ground, my son wanted to get back what he thought was a present, which was our daughter's remains in a ribbon-wrapped box. Jude helped me put dirt on top of the box.

In our times of pain, I am reminded of Lamentations 1:12, which is often used in the Stations of the Cross and which clearly foreshadows Our Lord's pain: "Is it nothing to you, all you who pass by? Look and see if there is any sorrow like my sorrow." Sometimes, as my wife and I went through our miscarriage, we grieved together while friends and family seemed to merrily move along with their lives, many of them never experiencing this sorrow. When I opened up to others about my miscarriage, many didn't say anything. Did anyone understand? It made me feel frustrated at their insensitivity. On a few occasions, while driving home from work, I would cry out to God in tears, "I want my child!" Seeing women with pregnant bellies had been the most glorious sight, but now there was some pain, for it reminded me of what we had lost. At times I was frustrated with God. My wife told me she was angry at God, and her outlook on pregnancy has been destroyed. I think this is a normal reaction.

Six months after Angelica's death and less than two months from her due date, a close priest friend told me, "It is time to move on," which hurt deeply. In my heart I said, "Father, forgive them; for they know not what they do" (Luke 23:34). Anyone who has lost a child knows you just don't move on, especially when you have not grieved properly for them. Losing a child leaves a scar that does not heal in this life, because once a new soul is created, it lives forever.

The following day, I sent the priest an email reminding him that most abortions occur near the same time most women have a miscarriage, which is during the first trimester. I told him that a woman who has an abortion never fully moves on. While we try to move on from the child we desperately wanted, a part of us has died, and the pain will always be there. We will not be downcast forever, we will find joy again, but what the world misses is that miscarriage is a big deal. Above all, we have the hope, God willing, that if we persevere, we will be reunited with them in the Nursery of Heaven.

For many, having another baby provides the healing remedy, but you cannot always count on that baby coming. Instead, we must hold on to the truth that God knows what He is doing. God is good, even when we do not understand His plan. If God blesses us with another child, I know our hearts will be filled with even greater gratitude and tears. If not, we must trust Him, for He knows what is best.

When my wife and I made our marriage vows before God, we never pictured so much suffering so early on. When you remain open to God's will, suffering is inevitable. I have suffered from seeing large families at Mass, having friends proudly declare that their wives were pregnant, receiving texts containing pictures of my friends' babies and pregnant wives, learning that some Catholic friends were unabashedly becoming pregnant through immoral means of conception such as IVF or IUI (intrauterine insemination), and hearing that my wife's lesbian classmate was having a baby. When people tell me that they are done having children or are spacing their children because it is a little hectic around the house, I feel a thorn in my side. I think to myself, "*It must be nice to tell God your plans.*" Seeing my son play by himself when he ought to be chasing his little brother or sister around has ripped me to the core. Above all, I have suffered the most from seeing my beautiful wife lie in bed many nights with tears in her eyes. I have often cried out to God, "Have mercy on us, but especially my wife." As most men do, I have wanted to "fix" a situation for which there is no simple solution.

With God's grace and the counsel of a holy priest, I am resigning myself to God's will and hopefully embracing it. I do not always understand it, but I have found joy in the cross because Our Lord suffers with me. Suffering has opened me to other friends who have not been so fortunate to have even one living child. Each of us has our own crosses. In devout Catholic circles, there can be an unhealthy competition to see who can have the biggest family. We should not view our children as trophies but as gifts from God.

When I meet someone who has lost a child, I am no longer indifferent to their pain; it causes me to choke up. I want to let them know I have been down to Calvary twice before, and I cannot let them carry their cross alone. Perhaps if we had the ten children that my wife and I dreamed about, without ever experiencing a child loss, I wouldn't have been able to enter into the pain of my brothers and sisters. Perhaps if we never lost a child, we wouldn't long for Heaven as much as we do now.

After losing our precious babies, I have also become even more passionate about the unborn child, who is the greatest gift and yet most vulnerable person in our society. In a mysterious way, losing two children has drawn me into a deeper union with God the Father and with the Mother of Sorrows — both lost their Son, only to find Him again. And my hope is this: what was once lost will be found again in the "resurrection of the body, and life everlasting," as the Apostles' Creed proclaims. God willing, I long to be reunited with my children in Heaven and see their beautiful faces. Faces I so longed to gaze on at their birth. Little hands and feet I longed to touch. Even if I do not recognize them at first, I will look for their sign, kind of like the one my wife made with Jude when she was pregnant with Thomas. Perhaps this time the Blessed Mother will assist them, and it will read like this: "Daddy, we are Thomas John and Angelica Rose. We missed you." In the meantime, I will seek their prayers, so that one day we will be together for all eternity praising God. Though the world will never know Thomas and Angelica, I know them, and they will live on forever in our hearts.

CHAPTER 5

Miscarriage

Two Years of Winter

Amanda O'Hearn

It was two years ago that I had my first miscarriage.[31] We had just returned from my brother's wedding in Wisconsin, which included a weeklong family vacation in Duluth. Although it was early, I shared the news that I was pregnant. It was a time of joy, hope, and excitement for the future. My sister Esther returned to North Carolina with us for a week's visit. My sister, my twenty-month-old son, Jude, and I looked forward to doing many fun activities and making new memories while my husband was at work. Five days into Esther's visit, on June 22, 2017, I started cramping and bleeding. I was completely stunned and shocked.

We decided to get an ultrasound two days later. I was so grateful that my sister was with me and could stay home with Jude. When Patrick and I arrived at the pregnancy center, they were having Mass in one of the conference rooms, so we attended. It was probably the most difficult Mass I have ever sat through, as I tried to keep my tears wiped and not to sniffle too loud.

[31] This manuscript was first completed in 2019. Two years of winter turned into six years year of winter before God would bless Amanda and Patrick with another child.

Following Mass, I was escorted into the ultrasound room by myself. That was their policy. At the time, I did not mind, because I so badly wanted to see what was going on. I told the doctor I thought I was nine or ten weeks along. When she started scanning, she didn't say anything. She just kept looking and searching. All I knew is that I didn't see what would look like a nine-week baby. Then she finally said, "Okay, Amanda, here is the gestational sac. This is definitely not what we would expect to see at nine weeks. This is more what we would expect to see just before six weeks, with no yolk sac yet visible." I went to the pregnancy center knowing that something was wrong, and we left that day unclear as to whether I had had a miscarriage. I felt that there was little hope, but my husband, Patrick, continued to pray for a miracle.

I know now that it was likely a blighted ovum, and all we were seeing was the empty gestational sac. A few days later, I returned alone to see if there was any forward progress, but I knew it was a miscarriage because I had continued to bleed. What we found was an even smaller gestational sac, so it was confirmed: I was miscarrying our baby. We will never know whether I was really six or nine weeks. The doctor said there was no obvious cause — just "genetics," as they say. My husband and I still do not know why we miscarried. It was likely a genetic issue that prevented the baby from forming properly, which I accepted.

My mother had two miscarriages before giving birth to me and then two others later. I knew it could happen, but I never thought it would happen to me. Nothing can prepare you. I was mildly consoled by the fact that a certain percentage of pregnancies end in a miscarriage for no known reason. There was nothing wrong that the doctors could find, and I was relieved by this. After crying for a while after the second ultrasound, Esther and I took Jude to the park. It seems like an odd thing to do, but in my grief I realized that sometimes it is okay to pretend your life is normal by visiting familiar places and people. No one would know that I just miscarried by looking at me. I would be safe.

I was disappointed that my sister's visit, which was supposed to be fun and memorable, was bombarded by such earth-shattering sadness due to our baby's death. Esther was also there when we buried the remains of our miscarried baby at our parish cemetery. Grateful for Esther's support, I was also saddened that my teenage sister had to witness such sorrow.

In grief, I am reminded that we are human, and our emotions are often unexpected, uncontrollable, yet very real. What I have learned is that you need to allow yourself to feel what you are feeling. If you hold it in, it is going to come back later even worse. Grief is normal and natural; it's perfectly human. We should not allow ourselves to feel guilty for feeling a certain way, as this is just a waste of mental energy.

We told some friends very early on that we were pregnant, only to tell them one month later that we had miscarried. Upon hearing the tragic news, they brought us a meal, which is a beautiful gesture for a grieving family. I was very grateful, but I also remember being angry. I didn't want a meal; I just wanted my baby! Then I felt guilty for feeling that way. I should just be grateful, right? Little did I know at the time that this was only the beginning of many conflicting feelings I would experience. It is a normal part of grief. Grief is the process you go through when trying to integrate the trauma of a loss into everyday life. It takes time because there is no area of your life left untouched. It cannot be processed all at once. This is why it comes in waves.

I remember getting ready to go to the cemetery. I wore a navy blue dress. One of my friends told me that when she miscarried, she collected her baby's remains the best she could and put them in a bag in the freezer. This is quite an alarming thought — to put your dead baby in the freezer until you can bury him — but that is what I did. It was my sweet child, after all — my baby. I would rather try to collect his little remains than let them go into a toilet, of all places. (If you have done that, please do not feel guilty. You can only do your best at the time.) I would rather bury our baby in the cemetery with an engraved stone and visit him. I believed it was the right thing to do, but sometimes I think this is the more difficult path.

I did not want to get in the car to go to the cemetery. I cried the whole way there and through the entire ceremony. I brought a whole box of tissues with me, because I knew I would need it. What I remember most about the ceremony is that the priest had my husband put dirt on top of the wooden box the baby was in. I remember thinking, Seriously?! You're going to make us put the dirt on top? I was shocked and horrified. I remember going to my grandfather's funeral a couple years previously. My brother commented on how crazy it was to see the hole dug and to see the dirt beneath the coffin. They did not lower him while people were still there weeping. I was shocked by the dirt. I already knew it, everyone knows it, but I was shocked by the fact that we had to put dirt on top of our baby and then just leave him there, cold and covered in dirt.

There were so many emotions that day. I was sad that we were burying our baby, that my fourteen-year-old sister was witnessing such a thing, that I couldn't even comfort my husband in his grief because I was so overwhelmed in mine. I was sad that my belly was not going to expand over the next nine months and I would have to put my maternity clothes away. I was sad because I was never going to meet my baby in this life, that I would never see him grow, that Jude had lost a sibling and wouldn't grow up with this baby. We named our baby Thomas John, after St. Thomas More and St. John the Baptist. We received a beautiful bouquet of white roses, and we had several supportive friends come to the ceremony, which was comforting.

Shortly after my sister went home, life tried to return to "normal" but it wouldn't. I started to sense this vast void inside of me. It was an indescribable sorrow. There had been a tiny being taking up space inside of me and starting to grow who was now gone. Emptiness took over my body, and most of all, my heart. I did not even have an ultrasound picture to look at to remind me of him. I had nothing special that was just his. In a way, it is beautiful, because he was so detached from this world that not a thing ever belonged to him, save my heart.

A few weeks later, we went walking with some dear friends at a nearby park. Their son is a little younger than Jude, so they were little buddies. During our visit, they informed us with great joy that they were expecting their second child. They had just found out, and our friend was only nine weeks along. They talked about their ultrasound and how everything "looked good." We were overjoyed, happy, and excited for them. But something hit us later that night after we got home. We both had the same thought at the same time: "Do you think they should have told us so soon after our miscarriage?" We had only buried our baby a few short weeks earlier. This was another example of the conflicting feelings I would continue to have for the next two years.

I was happy for my friend, but I was also feeling something else. It didn't take me long to calculate that since I was between six and nine weeks when I miscarried, we would have been due around the same time. The weeks went by, and I thought things would get a little better, but they only seemed to worsen. I was still crying all the time. It felt so unfair. I thought, "*Why did my baby die and not hers? Why am I left with an empty womb and on top of it I have to watch one of my best friends go through everything that I should be going through, too?*" I kept trying. I thought maybe this time I see her it will be okay. Maybe I am better now.

But every time I saw her, I felt sad and depressed. I would cry when I got home. I started to feel stuck, like nothing was helping me move forward in my grief. I was overjoyed for my friend's pregnancy and the promise new life brings, but her very joy, the sight of her growing belly, her glowing face, new maternity clothes, ultrasounds, preparations for the baby, were all a heart-wrenching reminder of what I had lost. I also grieved something new: that we wouldn't share our pregnancies and births in the same way. How exciting it would have been to have a baby at the same time as one of your dearest friends and watch the children grow up together!

Through therapy, I later came to understand that I was being triggered every time I saw her. It was such a tough place to be, because I wanted to see my friend and share in her joy, but seeing her meant I was going to go home crying again. At one point, I avoided seeing her for a month. This helped a little. But when I saw her again, my guard went up and the tears came back on the way home.

I was invited to her baby shower, but I told her I just couldn't come. She understood. But I did not understand why God was torturing me like this. I loved babies and everything having to do with them, but now seeing them or going to a baby shower or walking by the baby section at the store was a torment, and I had to avoid it or my eyes would flood with tears as I tried to hold it together long enough to get to the car, where I could let it all out.

I kept thinking that maybe I would be pregnant again soon, but it seemed like it was never going to happen. Month after month rolled by and my would-be due date came around — and I still wasn't pregnant. This was the most difficult part of losing my little Thomas, besides the shock in the beginning: the approaching due date for me and my friend, which would result in very different outcomes. My friend had a beautiful baby girl, and my arms were still empty and my belly was still flat. I think the single most difficult moment was when she sent me a picture of her introducing the baby to her son. I never knew joy and pain could be so intermingled and so intense. I sobbed uncontrollably for quite a while, and I felt like something deep inside of me died right then.

Many nights in the weeks and months after losing Thomas, I would lie with Jude until he fell asleep. I would cuddle with him and hold him, and I would cry and cry. I was so grateful that God had given me one child I could hold and love. I have thanked God a thousand times for him after losing Thomas. Jude was oblivious to the loss, so he was always his joyful, happy self.

I kept thinking that my grief would get easier after my friend's baby was born, but in reality, her baby was still a painful reminder of who should have been in my arms too. Then I thought that maybe after the one-year anniversary it would get better, but it didn't. At that time, literally all the moms in my friend group had their second baby, and I just couldn't take it anymore. It was difficult to go to Mass and see them because I was reminded of what I lost and what I so deeply longed for. This longing was so deep it hurt. In their presence the void in my life felt tangible. It was so painful and sad. And it was out of my control. I couldn't just wish it away or simply decide that I was going to be happy now.

Every time I saw my pregnant friends, I was triggered in my grief. After much thought and prayer, we switched parishes. I was torn over this decision, but I knew we had to do it. I had to find a few "safe places" where I would not be triggered in my grief. I could still be friends with them — they did nothing wrong, after all — but I did not need the weekly reminder of how we still didn't have another baby and everyone else's families were growing. We had several people ask if Jude was our "*only one*" or if I was pregnant, which was hurtful and insensitive, especially on Mother's Day of all days.

The difficulties continued for the next few months. We received many different pregnancy and birth announcements from friends. I tried to find Scripture verses that spoke to me, but mostly I still felt crushed in grief. I reached a low point after my friend had her baby. I was miserable and unhappy. I was depressed and weary. I may have started to experience adrenal fatigue, and I think it started to affect my thyroid. I was unable to sleep well at night, and when I woke up I didn't feel rested. I felt like a dark cloud was above my head. I was irritable all the time, and I was not able to laugh anymore and nothing seemed to help. I didn't like the person I was becoming. I felt like I had to get used to the "new me," which wasn't a good me.

Patrick said he just wanted me to be joyful again. I did too. But I had no idea how to make that happen. I felt swallowed up, like I was in a boat on a raging sea, holding on for dear life waiting for the storm to pass, but there was no end in sight. Looking back now, my under-functioning thyroid was a factor in my terrible mood and my inability to move forward. People often feel miserable with just an underactive thyroid and I had that combined with a miscarriage and a difficult situation with my friend. I struggled greatly with all of this for a long time.

This is when I knew I needed help, and my husband helped me to admit it. I needed emotional help from a therapist and to see an ob-gyn, because it had been a year and I still wasn't pregnant. In July 2018, I found a great Catholic therapist and a great Catholic ob-gyn. I started doing Eye Movement Desensitization and Reprocessing (EMDR) with the therapist, a technique used for many different types of traumas that aids in the healing process by reducing your emotional response to different triggers. You create a new, positive neuropathway in your brain — you think of a happy memory or place or remember an old one and then you talk about the situations or memories that trigger you while thinking of your happy place and looking at a series of flashing lights. The result is that your response is calmed down, so you can better handle those situations in the future, whether they arise in your mind or in person. Although things were still difficult, this therapy aided me on the path to healing.

In July, I also went to see the ob-gyn. I was very excited about this practice because their method for solving problems is not birth control or in vitro fertilization (IVF). I knew my body could grow a healthy baby. I just needed some healing. Since my thyroid stimulating hormone (TSH) was too high, I wanted to get it checked again, because I had found out three months earlier that my TSH was elevated to 7.0. I had been doing a thyroid-healing diet to try to avoid medication. We did some blood work, and I had hopes it was going to improve because I didn't feel any worse physically.

On August 3, I took a pregnancy test because I had been a little nauseous. To my absolute shock, it was positive! I didn't know what to do! It had been a little over a year since my miscarriage. I knew I needed to find out what my TSH was, because I knew that could be a factor in miscarriage. I was searching for the number to call the doctor and explain everything when my phone rang and it was her! I thought, "*Oh my goodness, I'm so glad you called! But wait, why did you call? Oh, the blood work!*" She was calling because my TSH had risen to 12.9, which is outrageously high. The connection was not very good, and I kept losing her during the conversation. I told her that I had taken a pregnancy test and was pregnant probably six times before she heard me. It felt so ironic and hilarious. She told me that a normal range for pre-conception for TSH would be below 2.5, and that she was going to put me on Nature-Throid, a pig thyroid hormone. She said we would do a six-week ultrasound in a couple of weeks and that I should go get my HCG and progesterone tested that day.

When the hormone tests came back "excellent," I felt much better, and being on the medication made me feel more at ease too. I felt like this pregnancy was going to go better. I knew hypothyroidism is associated with infertility, so I asked the doctor how it was possible to get pregnant with such an elevated TSH. She told me that it is not impossible but that she knew of patients who had lost a baby when their TSH was elevated. Other than that, she didn't extend any special caution or tell me not to get my hopes up.

I was so excited to be pregnant! It felt like we had waited an eternity for this baby and it was finally here. I quickly realized it was both *exciting* and *scary* to be pregnant after losing a baby. I had mild PTSD from losing Thomas. I remember being anxious every time I went to the bathroom because I was afraid I was going to see blood. So I checked all the time.

A couple of weeks later, at my six-week ultrasound, I found that I was seven weeks along and the baby was measuring six weeks with a heart rate at 88 bpm. My doctor said the normal heart rate was 90–120 bpm for the gestational age the baby was. She said that could be normal and we might just be a little off with the dates. I was to come back next week for another ultrasound to make sure everything was progressing properly. The ultrasound tech told me congratulations, and I started to feel happy again. I felt like everything was working out great and it was going to be okay this time.

I remember getting so excited, and Patrick was as well. I started digging out my maternity clothes just to look at them, even though I surely didn't need them yet. I started letting myself dream and hope. I prayed specifically that God would have mercy on me and let my baby live. Although I wasn't given a due date yet, I knew this was going to be an Easter baby and I was so excited because it was close to my birthday and my mother's birthday.

At my ultrasound the following week, the nurse took my vitals and said, "I know this is a sensitive appointment, right? So we are going to take good care of you." I remember thinking that she was nuts and everything was going to be fine. Yes, I had a miscarriage once, but it was not going to happen again. I was on medication for my thyroid, and I felt fine so everything would be fine. The doctor performed the ultrasound this time and it was set up so that I couldn't see the screen; I was facing the doctor.

She started scanning and she was smiling. And then her smile faded and her face became serious. I thought, "*Oh, no! Why was I looking at her? Just look at the ceiling, maybe it's okay, she hasn't said anything yet.*" Then she said that she didn't see any cardiac activity. I held my breath and thought, "*Just wait, it's going to pop up on the screen, you just didn't pick it up yet.*" She kept scanning and looking and she said the baby was still measuring six weeks, and that is when I realized it was true. This baby has died too. My first thought was, "*Oh God, why couldn't you have mercy on me, just this once?*" I was instantly angry with God. How could He let this happen? He could have stopped it easily. And after all the suffering I have already been through with the first one.

I was completely dumbfounded. My baby had died sometime in the previous week without my knowing it. Wouldn't I have a feeling that this was going to happen? As a mother, wouldn't I have some idea, some intuition? But I didn't; I was completely clueless. I had thought that miscarriage would happen to me once but not again. I was on to greener pastures now, wasn't I? This can't happen twice in a row!

I had naively gone to this ultrasound without Patrick again, (Jude came along) thinking everything would be fine, and I found out the horrible news alone. I ended up calling him when I got to the car. We decided to just carry on with our day and would start grieving together later that night. We had been through this before, and I wasn't even bleeding or cramping yet. This was called a "missed miscarriage."

A few minutes after leaving I was pulled over for speeding in a school zone. It was probably the worst day of my life. It was 9:40 a.m. when I got pulled over, no kids in sight, and everyone was speeding through there. It wasn't an area I normally drove in. And I got singled out. "*Such is my luck,*" I thought. In my grief, shock, and anger I almost laughed at the situation. Nothing could have made me feel worse at that moment, after finding out that the baby still inside me was dead. I didn't even care what kind of ticket he gave me or how much it was going to cost. The only thing that would have upset me is if I had gotten arrested. Pretty sure I hadn't done anything to warrant that, I rolled down the window and took off my sunglasses, revealing my tears and red eyes. In the end, the officer did not give me a ticket, and there was God's mercy, but I thought it was very misplaced that morning. I would rather have had the four-hundred-dollar ticket and a living baby in my womb.

After I got my "warning" and the police officer gave Jude a sticker, we went to our chiropractor. This is where I was planning to go anyway, and I decided that I might as well stop since I had let him know I was pregnant. The doctor's first words were, apologetically, "You're not in charge." And I thought to myself, "*Yes, this man 'gets' it.*" I'm not in charge, God is in charge, and even though this is a horrible situation to be in, God is there. I called my mom on the way home and she had hopeful words for me, reminding me that she had two miscarriages before me and saying, "You never know, maybe you'll have a whole pack of kids yet."

We had a beach trip planned with most of my family and Patrick's parents. This trip was a big deal because my family had never made a trip to North Carolina like this and most of them had never seen the ocean. I was going to be eleven or twelve weeks pregnant, and I thought maybe I would start to show by then. To make a bad situation worse, I ended up carrying the baby for three more weeks after the ultrasound appointment, and Hurricane Florence decided to show up right before our beach trip. A miscarriage, a hurricane, and family visiting are quite a horrible combination indeed! We ended up being able to find another beach house that had minimal damage from the hurricane. While I was happy that our dream family vacation was not ruined, I was crippled by grief again. I couldn't even go in the water because I was still bleeding.

Conflicting feelings seem to be a recurring theme of my life. Sometimes, I just don't understand what God is thinking! All I know is that His grace seems to be enough, along with lots of tears and a supportive husband. That is how I got through it, and how I am still getting through it. There are still days when I get triggered by something, and I feel crushed with grief. There are also days when I feel like I am doing okay. If my thyroid function ever balances out, maybe I will even feel good again.

We ended up burying our second miscarried baby next to her miscarried brother. We didn't invite any friends or family. It was just us three, Patrick, Jude, and me, and a wonderfully understanding and compassionate priest. I knew right after I found out about this baby that I was going to dread the burial ceremony. I knew how hard it was from the first time. For some reason this was harder for me because we knew this baby was a girl. With Jude, I had a dream of a baby boy around the time of conception. With Thomas, I had a dream of a baby boy when I was miscarrying. With Angelica Rose, I had a dream of a baby girl when I miscarried. I take those dreams as signs from God.

We decided to use our own box for Angelica's coffin, and I wrapped it in a bunch of white and pink ribbons that were on the purity candle that Patrick lit on our wedding night and tied them in a bow. God didn't allow me the opportunity to tie ribbons in her hair, but I made sure I tied them around her little coffin. When I think of Angelica's ceremony, I think of that beautiful ribbon-wrapped box being covered in dirt. I was struck by the dirt at her ceremony as well. On the way to the cemetery, Jude held the box and he said it was a present. He didn't understand when we put the box in the ground and started to cover it. It was completely heartbreaking. Eventually,

Patrick convinced him to help put the dirt on top. By the time the ceremony concluded, we could see a beautiful sunset through the trees. I took the sunset that night of Angelica's burial as a sign of God's love and presence in our grief.

I often wonder what God is trying to teach me in my loss and grief. Perhaps He is teaching me patience, compassion, trust, hope, and surrender. I wonder how God is going to redeem pregnancy for me because I hate ultrasounds now, and although I long for a baby, I am afraid to be pregnant again. Babies are not a cheerful sight for me. They make me sad and I hate feeling that way, but I cannot control it. I also wonder how God will redeem my relationship with my friend. For now, we have agreed not to see each other, and I think there is wisdom in that. I don't know how long this friend break will be. It may be for quite a long time, but it is impossible to heal when the bandage keeps getting ripped off. It is very difficult not to see my dear friend, but I know that I must protect my heart. It breaks my heart when Jude says, "Can we go see them?" and I have to say, with tears in my eyes, "No, maybe another time, sweetie." I want to see them too, but I know it will hurt, and the conflicting feelings will surface again. They say that time heals all wounds, but I think really they should say, "God heals all wounds in time." This healing will not happen, though, unless we are open to God's grace.

The real pain is not right after the miscarriage, as difficult as that is, but when everyone stops sending cards, bringing meals, and asking how you are. When I lost all those supports, it became even more trying for me. I wanted to return to "normal life," but I found out there is no "normal" anymore because my baby has died. In grief, one has to find a new normal. The world marches on, but I have not marched on, because I am forever changed.

I remember sitting in my college embryology class discussing the intricate set of events that must occur for a baby to be conceived, grow, and develop. During the professor's lecture on the complex cell signaling and tissue differentiation, he paused and said something that I will never forget: at the moment of conception, the whole universe is changed forever. I see now what a beautiful truth this is, because God has created a unique and unrepeatable precious being. And this little being is mine. He has my and my husband's DNA. He or she is uniquely our child.

We have one beautiful son on earth, and we have two baby saints in Heaven. In moments of sadness, we remind ourselves that they are in Mary's arms in the presence of the saints and angels. Over five years of marriage, we have experienced the pain and sorrow of the Passion, and we are still waiting for our resurrection, for our spring to come. We are praying and trusting that it will happen in God's time. If we do have another baby, it will be a double rainbow baby.

Something that helped me was journaling my thoughts and feelings. After I miscarried, I had an image of myself as a rose trampled underfoot or covered in snowdrifts. When I was ready, I would be a bud waiting for pregnancy, and then I would bloom when I found out I was pregnant. Then, when I miscarried, I had an image of the rose being cut off and stomped on, then buried in snowdrifts again. I prayed that God would help me to bear the loss and grief and to bring back the sunshine. When I am ready, I will ask Him to let me bloom again, because although there is risk of another loss, it is worth it. I have a deep, soulful longing for spring, but I fear it for its risks.

Eliminating my triggers and finding safe places that wouldn't predictably cause tears, sadness, and terrible thoughts have really helped. This can mean many different things, depending on your situation. I also allowed myself more "me time": walking in nature, listening to music (especially Audrey Assad), having girls' nights, watching a movie with my husband, talking to my sister on the phone, and finding a way to laugh again. I cultivated new hobbies like crocheting, calligraphy, fermenting sauerkraut, and starting a book club, and revived old hobbies like gardening and card making. I also cut back on my job as a nanny. A miscarriage is a great shock to the body, mind, and soul, so you need to find ways to nourish and replenish all of those.

Ten months after losing Angelica, I was surprised by a memory of the moment when I saw her sweet little heart beating on the ultrasound — surprised with joy! I was shocked because until now, all the memories I had of her or Thomas were painful ones. This is a sign of healing and this is why we grieve — to remember without all the pain. It is nothing but a grace to experience this, and we must look forward to the day we can see their short lives for the light that they are and not as traumatic experiences. That memory was the beginning of a time of peace for me. This trial is still difficult, but I also have some sense of peace with my losses, and this is completely new to me. I don't think I will ever come to a point in this life where I can say, "I am healed," but I will come to a point where I can say, "I am okay."

We must be patient in healing; it does not happen overnight as we would like, but little by little we may see the snow melt. And in time, we may be surprised by a bud that blossoms into a fragrant, captivating flower. My prayer is that God will heal us in His time, if we remain open to His love and grace.

CHAPTER 6

MISCARRIAGE

His Name Is Sam

Sue McIlroy

IT WAS A COLD January morning, right after the New Year. I was snuggling with my husband, Bob, and he was aimlessly flipping through the channels with the remote. It was our routine. He would flip, and I would get frustrated. I never like what he puts on, but if I finally start to get interested . . . he flips. That morning he flipped from thriller to comedy to music, then back to thriller. The show he momentarily stopped at caught my attention. There was a woman named Telly, played by Julianne Moore, and she was searching for her son. She frantically asked everyone she knew, "Do you know where my son is? Do you remember him?" Everyone thought she was crazy and responded, "Who are you talking about? We don't know him. What's wrong with you? He never existed!"

As my husband began to flip to the next channel, I told him to stop, and that I wanted to watch the rest of the movie. I was curious about what happened to Telly's son. I wondered if the movie was about a government conspiracy or about some alien thing. Little did I know that the movie was about something more profound — at least for me.

In the last few minutes of the movie, Telly encounters a strange man who knows the answers to her questions. However, this man wants to erase all her memories of her son and challenges her to give him the last memory she had, which was the day she gave birth to him. The man succeeds in erasing her memory, and to prove that he has succeeded, he asks her, "That boy. What was his name?"

Telly responds, "What boy?" At this point, the movie flashes back to her memories of her pregnancy, before she ever held her son. She rubs her belly and says, "I had life inside me. I had life. I have a child. I have a son. I . . . have a son. His name is Sam."

I was not prepared for these words. They pierced me to the core of my being, and without warning, I cried tears that I didn't know I had, and these tears flowed without ceasing. This movie was supposed to be another one of those typical ridiculous movies we watched on Saturday mornings. How was this movie able to reach the buried pain that I had been struggling with for the past year and a half, and how was it able to express so much truth in such few words? When I asked Bob what the name of the movie was, he replied, *The Forgotten*. Upon hearing the title, I cried and sobbed even more. For I had a child whom we "lost" through miscarriage, and his name was Sam. Because of this miscarriage, Bob, Sam, and I were made members of the club, the Forgotten and the Forsaken. This is a club filled with many moms, dads, and babies that I never knew existed until we lost our baby. It is a club that doesn't advertise, yet its members are many who are mourning in silence and are living a silent sorrow.

My story of silent sorrow began on May 13, 2017, the one hundredth anniversary of Our Lady's first appearance in Fatima. It was a beautiful sunny day. The sun's rays were shining through the stained-glass windows of our church upon the altar, where my family and I were standing with other families about to sign "Our Consecration to

Mary." As my friend signed her consecration, I clearly remember thinking how beautiful she was because she was blessed. Her tummy was starting to show the baby they were preparing to welcome in August. Little did I know that I was also blessed with a child in my womb as I stood at the altar alongside her.

At age forty-seven, I thought that my life of childbearing was over. My youngest daughter, Hannah, was five, and in the time since she was born, I had been experiencing all the lovely signs of perimenopause/menopause. The Lord had already blessed me with eight children, seven of whom were miracles that we were told we would never have because of medical problems. However, God healed me and blessed us with eight children. After Hannah's birth and realizing that my season to bear children was ending, I went through a grieving process and finally put that part of my life on the shelf.

The day after the Marian consecration was Mother's Day. While cleaning, I found a box of unused pregnancy tests. Ironically, I hadn't had a cycle for a while, and I was feeling tired. Convinced that I was officially at the beginning of menopause, I took a test, thinking that it would be negative. A positive result was the furthest thing from my mind. So when the line on the test turned pink, I thought, "Oh my! How in the world can this be?"

Because of my past struggles with high-risk pregnancies, I called the doctor right away. He told us to come in immediately for an ultrasound to make sure everything was okay and to confirm that the pregnancy wasn't ectopic. When the doctor did the ultrasound, he confirmed that I was pregnant but was unable to confirm the location of my baby. He called it a "pregnancy of unknown location." Because my doctor was also concerned with the results of my blood work, he said that I needed to come in for another ultrasound that Friday, and if he saw that I had an ectopic pregnancy, he would have me go into surgery right away.

I cannot convey the sadness and sorrow I felt and the fear I had while waiting for the upcoming ultrasound. I didn't understand why they didn't know where my baby was. I didn't know how to pray—should I pray for a struggling baby in my womb or to a baby that has already passed and was with God in Heaven? I pleaded with Jesus, the Good Shepherd, to find our baby, to bring him or her home, and to let us know where he or she was. I knew that God could grant a miracle if He desired, but I felt like the centurion in the Gospel. Who am I to ask for such a gift, for I am so unworthy? But I prayed anyway: "Lord, I am so unworthy for You to enter under the roof of my womb, but only say the word, and I and my baby shall be healed!"

On the day of our ultrasound, I was nervous. When the technician did the test, she found our baby right away. He was alive! He was where he was supposed to be—in my womb. The ultrasound screen showed the sound waves of a repetitive heartbeat. Our baby's heart was beating, and the sound of his life was breathlessly beautiful.

To hear life, to hear our baby at such a young age, was a gift, a miraculous gift. With our own eyes and ears, we saw and heard his life beat, "I'm here ... I'm here ... I'm here ... I am alive!"

When I looked over at Bob, his eyes were filled with tears and he began to cry, a cry of relief. Then Bob looked at me and said with a bold faith, "Sue, this baby is special. He is going to do something to change the world." When Bob spoke these words, I believed in my heart of hearts that he was speaking truth, and I had hope and peace that all was going to be well with our baby.

On Monday morning, I went to Mass to praise and thank God for the miracle he gave us. As I was leaving, a lady congratulated me and ended her greeting saying, "Jesus, I trust in You." Little did I know how much I would need these words, because my hope was to be tested again.

Shortly after, my doctor called and said that he was still concerned about my pregnancy because my HGC levels were low. He wanted me to do more tests and to come in for a second ultrasound later in the week.

So, I started the prayer ritual again and continued to cling to Jesus by going to daily Mass, receiving the Eucharist, and pleading with Him using the words of the centurion. One morning at Mass, another lady stopped me and asked me some questions. In response, I told her that I had complete confidence in God that He could heal and save our baby if He willed it. I told her that I was praying the centurion's prayer.

Surprisingly, she responded that I was praying wrong. Because she is an incredible woman of faith whom everyone holds in high regard, I was taken aback and tried to explain my prayer. However, she repeatedly told me that I was praying wrong. She insisted that I needed to pray for God's will.

I was deeply hurt and confused by this encounter. I was a mother who was scared to death of losing my baby, and I was baring my heart to Jesus to save him. Any mother would plead for her child, wouldn't she? Even Mother Mary? We all know that Mother Mary was willing to do God's will and accept it. But she is a mother, and wouldn't she plead for Jesus so that He didn't have to suffer or die?

The encounter with this lady of faith put me in a spiritual quandary. For the next week or so, I struggled deeply with God on how to pray for my baby. I wanted to pray "the right way." So, when I tried to pray for God's will as the lady insisted, I felt like I was not being a good mother. When I prayed that Jesus would save my baby, I felt that I was dishonoring God by not praying for His will. These battling prayers and what seemed to be conflicting desires of my heart were a spiritual torment and continued for days.

When I finally had the second ultrasound, our baby was still alive. The doctor exclaimed how surprised he was and that there were many things throughout his years of practice that he couldn't explain and this was one of them. He was so confident that he gave us permission to leave the next day on our two-week family vacation.

During this vacation to the Outer Banks, which we look forward to every year, I was not present with my family in mind or body. I was completely distracted by the uncertainty of whether my baby would die and what I would do if something happened so many miles away from my home and my doctor. I wasn't as active as I usually was on vacation. After a week, I started to spot. Seeing this slight blood caused me to panic, to isolate myself from my family, and to struggle to pray to God.

When I asked my husband, who is a faithful man, to pray for our baby, he surprisingly scoffed and said that I was being ridiculous and that everything was going to be okay. He irritatingly said that I needed to trust in God. I sadly wondered, "What does my desire for prayer have to do with a lack of trust?" I felt rejected and alone, and I was angry that the man who prays for and with others was unable to pray with me, his wife, on behalf of our child. His response, along with the faithful lady's response at church, put me in a tailspin as I continued to struggle with praying.

Before we left to return home, we went to Confession and Mass. Distraught, I told a Franciscan priest everything about my fears regarding our baby and what the lady had said. He comforted me and said that the woman was in error and that our whole Catholic Faith, including our Mass, was based on intercessory prayer. He said that as the mom it was only right and natural to plead for my baby, and that I needed to go before Jesus right away and do so. And that is what I did. When I left the confessional, I was relieved to have permission to continue to pray for my baby as I so strongly desired to do from the beginning. Kneeling before Jesus, I felt my body relax and my tension leave, and in my moment of pleading, I was at peace. And yet, I also somehow knew that all was not well.

As we began our twelve-hour trip home, everything was okay. However, when we stopped for lunch, I discovered bright red blood when I used the restroom. I was not prepared for this. Continuing home, I started bleeding more and having contractions. We still had six hours to go before arriving home, and panic set in. I still had hope that my baby could survive and continued to pray for his life. We were driving through the Allegheny Mountains. Despite their vast size and imposing nature, they looked so small to me. Jesus' words, "If you have faith as a grain of mustard seed, you will say to this mountain, 'Move from hence to yonder place,' and it will move; and nothing will be impossible to you" (Matt. 17:20), resounded in my heart. The mountains seemed insignificant. I knew that the Lord could move them, and I knew he could save my baby. I begged Our Lord, reminding Him of this Scripture, and the entire trip home, I begged all the angels and all the saints to intercede for my baby, and I believed.

As my bleeding got heavier and the contractions became more intense, fear overcame me. All I wanted to do was get home, and we still had a very long way to go. I cried and panicked in the passenger seat. Being neither patient nor sympathetic, or so it seemed to me, Bob yelled that I needed to calm down and that there was nothing he could do. Unknowingly, bitterness toward my husband took root in my heart in those moments.

When we finally got home, I ran upstairs to my room. My husband went into his work mode and unpacked the van and tried to take care of work responsibilities. I felt so alone. My children would periodically knock on my door and hesitantly ask in a worried tone, "Mom, are you okay?" My husband never came.

Unexpectedly, my sister Sharon called me. She said she just wanted to see how I was doing. I cried and told her that I thought I was losing my baby. I was in so much pain, physically and emotionally, that I was barely able to get the words out. Sharon said that based on what she was hearing, she was convinced I was in labor and in the process of having a miscarriage. I had no clue that when someone miscarried their baby they went through the labor process. Sharon stayed on the phone with me, timing my contractions, talking me through the pain, and trying to calm me down. My sister knew my pain, a pain that I never realized until then, because she herself had five of her own miscarriages. Sharon stayed with me for hours and helped me to carry my pain. It was horrible, but as horrible as it was, I am so grateful that I felt it, because in experiencing that pain I was experiencing the life of my child, whom I would never get to hold.

Between my sister's coaching and my pain, I made multiple trips to the bathroom. I inspected everything that came out of me, because I was looking for my baby. I saved what I could, so that I could bring it to the doctor. As things became more intense, I cried the name of Jesus. I yelled His name, I pleaded His Name: "Jesus, Jesus! Jesus!!!" It was the only prayer I knew. People say that the name of Jesus is the most powerful prayer, and that when you say it, He is right beside you. But I did not feel His presence. I felt abandoned by Him. People also say that Jesus will answer your prayer when you call His name and that He will bring healing if you have faith. I had faith. But somehow, those promises were not meant for me, for I called upon the name of Jesus, pleading for my baby. I asked Jesus to save my baby, and He said no.

After hours of agony, the pain subsided at some point, and I fell asleep. When I woke up, it was morning, and all was calm and quiet. My sister called to check on me. When I told her that there was no more pain, she said that she thought it was over and that I needed to call my doctor.

When I did, the doctor told me to come in right away. I took everything that I had collected, because I wanted them to confirm that my baby was present. My husband, whose demeanor was much more calm and solemn, told me that he would take me. Before the doctor looked at what I brought, he did an ultrasound, and my husband was at my side.

I wasn't prepared for what I would see on the screen. I never really thought about it. When the technician scanned me, my baby appeared! He was so big and so beautiful and so much bigger than what I had seen two weeks earlier. I was surprised and so happy to see our baby, to see his increased size, and to see his precious form, that I did not fully comprehend what was happening. Then I heard my doctor say, "I am sorry, Susan. Your baby has no heartbeat."

In admiring how much my baby had grown and how beautiful he was, I never noticed that he was lifeless. I had no breath, and I had no thoughts. Our baby had died.

My doctor's only concern at that point was for me and my life. Because of all the blood I had already lost, he was worried about hemorrhaging and wanted me to have a dilation and curettage (D&C) right away. However, I wanted to have our baby naturally, and did not want to have a D&C, which I felt was harming my baby and causing him to be mutilated. I couldn't bear doing that to him. My doctor, husband, and family pleaded with me, because I had eight beautiful children to live for, and because of them, I agreed to do the surgery in two days.

When I went home, I started to prepare for the upcoming surgery. Because I had two friends who had buried their babies lost through miscarriage in our local Catholic cemetery, I wanted to see how I could save my baby's remains so I could bury Sam in the

Catholic cemetery as well. However, because my baby was younger gestationally, it would be difficult.

I did research and found an Ohio law, Senate Bill 175, entitled the Grieving Parents Act, which had been passed two years earlier and which said that parents had the right to claim their baby's remains if under twenty weeks. Prior to this law, the hospital had legal rights to what they considered "medical waste." I called the office of the senator where this bill originated. The legislative aide helped me and gave me advice on how to claim my baby's body. Although it is law, many people, medical personnel, and medical facilities are unaware of it and are not accustomed to returning the baby.

After learning my legal rights, I did what the legislative aide said and called my doctor and the hospital where the surgery was going to take place to tell them what I wanted. My doctor was very supportive and told me that he would do what he could, but that I needed to talk to the hospital. I called multiple people who passed me along to others when I told them that I wanted my baby returned to me after the procedure so I could bury him. Because there was no protocol for this, there was confusion. Eventually, a supervisor said that I needed to let the surgery center know when I went in and that I would have to sign a release.

When I went to the surgery center, I immediately told them that I had talked with a legislator and to the hospital staff and that I had permission to have my baby's remains. I asked for the paper to sign that would ensure this release. Since no one had ever requested their baby's return, they had a hard time getting the document.

When they took me back to prepare for the surgery, everyone was very kind, and some offered condolences, which surprised me because at that point I had not processed that I had a loss. Then my nurse came in and started talking about the procedure and mechanically said, "Oh, they gave me this paper for you to sign for the release of the specimen." Taken aback and confused, I hesitantly asked, "Are you talking about my baby?" Immediately, filled with regret, she apologized and said, "Yes, I'm talking about your baby."

While filling out the paper, I noticed that the release stated, "I have requested that the specimen or device be provided to me by. . . . " Seeing the word "specimen" in reference to my baby bothered me. I shyly crossed out the word specimen and wrote "baby" very lightly with pencil and in small print. I had to write "baby." I couldn't sign something that referred to my baby as a by-product. The same nurse who originally referred to my baby as a specimen noticed what I was doing and recognized my apprehension. Then she did the most beautiful thing. She took her black pen and wrote "BABY" in bold capital letters! Her seemingly insignificant act was a great gift of love, because she pronounced dignity on my baby. The nurse then promised me that she would advocate for my baby and make sure that everyone who encountered me or him before, during, and after the procedure knew to save my baby's remains so that I could bury him.

They wheeled me into the surgery room. I noticed the room looked exactly like the room where I had all my previous C-sections. I also saw my ob-gyn, who had delivered all my children. His face was somber and said it all: "This surgery is different." After "this" surgery, there would be no baby to hold. I started to cry, and they put me to sleep.

When I woke up, I was numb. The nurse told me that everything was set and that I should be able to get my baby's remains in twenty-four to forty-eight hours after it went to pathology. I was hoping that they would bring my baby to me right away so I could hold him. The need to hold my baby was so strong that my body physically yearned for him. Just as an amputee may feel his missing limb, I physically felt my baby missing from my womb. The hospital released me, and I went home.

Two days after the procedure, I asked for Sam's remains, but they said that I would have to call at the beginning of the following week.

When I did, I was told that I would have to wait another week. No one knew where my baby was or when I would get him back. This became another trauma for me. All I wanted was my baby and the chance to hold him. When I spoke with everyone, I was desperate and angry, but because I did not want them to discard my baby, I tried to be patient. I was at their mercy, and I didn't want them to do anything to hurt my baby. In addition to the anxiety of not knowing where Sam was, I was also hurt by the words they used to describe him. Almost every medical personnel would say, "Oh you mean 'the specimen,'" or "the medical waste," or "the products of conception." All these terms dehumanized my baby.

It was now two weeks since the surgery. Because it happened to be the feast of the Sacred Heart, I thought Jesus would help bring my baby back on this special day. However, when I called, still no one knew where my baby was. An administrator then told me that my baby wasn't even at the hospital and that they had shipped him downtown to the main campus. It would be another two weeks. I was angry and thought, "*How could they do this? How could God allow this?*" All I wanted was my baby back so I could hold him and give him a proper burial. I did everything I could to save my baby and his body.

Where was my baby? Where was my precious Sam? No one seemed to care where he was, not even Jesus. Mary Magdalene's desperation in not finding the body of Jesus became my experience. But I had no hope of resurrection. I only had visions of some high school teen chomping on his gum in the hospital basement accidentally throwing my baby away in the garbage. I had no control of the situation. I lost my baby. I lost him twice (first his life and now his body), and I didn't know where to find him.

A friend called me a short time after my phone call with the hospital. After I told her what happened, she called her dad, who was a pro-life advocate and had connections. He called me right away and said that he would help me and that he could get legal counsel to help me. Because I was afraid to cause problems, I was ambivalent. But he said that this was important and that I had every right to expect my baby back. His friend, who was a lawyer, called me the next day and said that he would help me. The lawyer instructed me to call a funeral home for help too, while he would contact the hospital administration to get action.

When I called the funeral home, I talked with a director who dealt with funerals for children and babies. He didn't know me; I was just a panicked mother calling him from out of the blue. When I told him my story, the funeral director was upset and said that I should have had my baby back within the twenty-four to forty-eight hours they had promised. He told me that I needed to call and demand my baby back. To which I responded, "But I don't know how? I need help." Without hesitancy, he spoke compassionately and in a powerful Italian accent said, "I'll help you. I'll get your baby back!"

For days, I had had no help and felt abandoned and forsaken. Within hours, the God who I thought had abandoned me brought me three strong, assertive men to help find my baby, a baby whom no one ever met and a baby whom no one would ever hold and see. These three men worked together to fight for my baby to have a final resting place.

Simultaneously, the lawyer called and drafted a letter for me, communicating with the top levels of the hospital, and the funeral director searched for my baby at the ground level. Within minutes, but after days and weeks of waiting, the funeral director called me and said that he had located my baby and that he was going to the hospital to get him. The baby had never even left the hospital. At the same time, the lawyer called and told me that the hospital administrators were going to release my baby's remains immediately. When I had lost hope, God intervened and moved the mountains for me. An hour later, the funeral director texted the most beautiful words I have ever read: "I have your baby, and he is safe in our care!"

The funeral director prepared Sam's remains for me and placed him in a beautiful gray marble urn. With the funeral director, the Catholic cemetery, and my pastor, I planned a Catholic burial service. Everything, including the grave and headstone, was generously given to us for free. Before the burial service, the funeral director allowed me to take my baby home in the urn for a few days so we could hold Sam and spend time with him. When I picked up Sam's remains from the funeral home, it was surreal. They brought Sam to me. I wrapped Sam, who was in an urn, in a baby blanket. I finally got to hold my baby whom I had yearned for. From the funeral home, I took Sam and a few of my children to our church, where I blessed him with holy water and placed him on the altar as a prayer of thanksgiving and consecration to Jesus. In the few days before the service, I held him in my arms and didn't let go. My husband noticed that I unconsciously rocked him and patted him like a newborn. It was my way of grieving. For the service, we had our children write letters to Sam and place them in the casket along with a baby rosary, a crucifix, a miniature statue of Mary, and part of the baby blanket that had cradled him. The service was beautiful and healing.

The days after losing and burying my baby were difficult ones. I went home and allowed myself to rest the next day, thinking I should be able to get back to my normal routine in a few days. Subconsciously, I thought everything was over, but it wasn't. The mourning was just beginning. My baby, whom we named Samuel Mary, Sam for short, had died, and I needed to face that. Because I was so wrapped up in pleading for my baby's life, searching for him, and doing all that I could for him to have a proper burial, I never processed anything. I had "lost" my baby and had a "miscarriage." These two words bothered me immensely because they did not convey the depth of my pain and my loss. For many years, when I heard that someone had a miscarriage, I was guilty of indifference and of thinking it was no big deal because it was a common occurrence. I never reflected on the suffering that was involved. The terms "miscarriage" and "lost my baby" somehow lessen the reality that a child has died. I didn't lose something meaningless like a tooth or a sock. I lost a child. My precious baby, my precious child, my precious Sam, had died.

Yet no one seemed to care, notice, or acknowledge this. A lady at my parish tragically lost her son in a car crash a few days before my baby died. Everyone, including me, was deeply saddened by this devastating accident. I prayed for her and offered up my sufferings for her and her son. I couldn't imagine the depth of her suffering. I struggled because I told myself that I had no "right" to mourn my situation because she had a son who died. I "only" had a miscarriage. But my flesh, my being, and my soul screamed, "My child died too!"

The silence and indifference were painful. This silence contributed to my feelings that I did not have a right to grieve or mourn. Many people never said a word, including some family members and close friends. I felt alone, forgotten, and forsaken. My loss was so deep, so real, so painful. All I wanted was a word, a word to release the pain so I could breathe — a simple, "How are you?" I wanted someone to reach out and touch my pain.

The comments of others further cemented my feelings that I didn't have a right to mourn and compounded my feelings of isolation. "You should be grateful. Why are you upset? You have eight children." In my grief, I was never ungrateful for the children I had; I was sad for the one who died. Many asked, "How many weeks was your baby?" This common and innocent question always pierced me. It was a question that I never wanted to answer, and it was a question that I had unfortunately asked of others when I had heard of their miscarriage. I hate this question because it is a question that "quantifies" the reality or the worth of my baby. Without fail, every time I answer it, people respond with a dismissive "Oh" and their face says, "That's all? That's not a big deal." As if to say, "Your baby wasn't real. Your loss isn't real. Your baby doesn't matter."

Others, in their attempt to make me feel better, said, "You should be grateful. Your baby probably had something wrong with it. Count your blessings." These comments also pierced me. I would have loved to care for my baby and would have done anything for him no matter what the disability or problem was. Taking care of him would have been a blessing, not a burden. I struggled with these comments because these people, who are pro-life warriors, tell mothers who are considering abortion that their children with disabilities have dignity and a right to life. So how can they dismiss the life of my baby who may have had the same disability but died through miscarriage? If we as Christians firmly teach and believe that life begins at the moment of conception, why wouldn't a mother mourn the child she never got to hold through the tragedy of miscarriage? If we don't mourn, acknowledge, and honor our babies who have died before they were born, how could we expect the mother who is considering an abortion to understand the sacredness and dignity of the child she is carrying?

Because of everything, I was hurt and bitter. I had bitterness toward others, such as the lady who corrected me for my prayer; my husband, who seemed not to care; the people who made insensitive comments; the close family members and friends who were indifferent; and even God, who seemed "asleep in the boat" during my storm. The physical, emotional, and spiritual pain was intense. To find rest, I found myself going to Confession quite often. In the confessional, God healed me and comforted me and took care of my wounds. A priest helped me to forgive those who hurt me. He challenged me to be honest with my husband about my feelings toward him. When I confronted him as the priest suggested, Bob sincerely expressed sorrow for his impatience and said that he reacted poorly because he was scared and sad too. The same priest apologized for all those who hurt me and asked for my forgiveness on their behalf. He told me that I needed to be honest with God about how I was feeling and that God didn't expect me to be stoic or "perfect" in my suffering. When I was leaving the confessional, he said, "Sue, remember that the 'right' prayer, the 'best' prayer, is always the one that comes from the heart." Another priest gave me the permission to mourn my baby. He firmly told me that because I was Sam's mom, that I not only had the "right" but also the "obligation" to mourn his passing. When this priest heard my whole story, he said, "Don't you see what was happening? Don't you see what God was doing? When you were looking for your baby, you were a witness to all those people. All they knew was that there was a mom who wanted her baby!" The life of Sam was a witness to others that no matter how hidden his life was and no matter how young he was, his life mattered and had dignity.

My desire to have people acknowledge that I lost a child, my determination to find his body, and my need to have permission to mourn Sam were all rooted in my quest to prove that Sam's life mattered and that he was a real person. One day, I received a sympathy card from a lady at church expressing her sorrow that Samuel Mary had passed away. In writing his name, she acknowledged him and that he was a person. It was a beautiful gift that gave me great comfort. One friend had his name and year written on a Christmas ornament, and another friend acknowledged his worth with a beautifully framed poem that expressed the dignity of his unborn life. These were beautiful gifts that brought me great comfort because they acknowledged the loss of my child and called Samuel by name.

I never realized the power and the beauty of a name. Our name shows personhood and dignity of life, a life worth remembering. Every year during the 3:00 p.m. service on Good Friday, our church acknowledges all the people who have passed away. On Good Friday, April 2018, my pastor read "Samuel Mary McIlroy" along with the other names of the deceased members of our church family. Hearing Sam's name proclaimed brought me so much peace and joy. I felt the Lord say, "Sam matters. His life counts just as these others do. I have called Sam by name. He is mine."

When God created Sam and put him in my womb, He called him by name. Sam's purpose and mission in life were hidden but were no less important than someone who lived to be a hundred. God called Sam home because he did what he was supposed to do though he was unknown. Although his life and worth are not quantified by the standards of this world, Sam's life is priceless and has dignity in the eyes of God. Although no one ever got to hear him cry, see him smile, or feel his embrace, his life forever impacts the life of his mom and family.

As much as I love Sam, I know that Sam loves us. He is in Heaven rooting for us, helping us, and comforting us. On his due date, I had an intense need to give birth, to be near my baby, and to hold him. It was a cold, snowy January day, and inches of fresh fallen snow blanketed the grass everywhere. I wanted to visit Sam at the cemetery but was hesitant because my friend had told me weeks earlier that the cemetery wanted people to do only roadside visits during the winter months so they wouldn't trip in the snow and get hurt. However, my need to be near my baby was overpowering. I wanted to lie down, to press my chest to and hold the ground where my baby was.

My baby's grave is in the back of the cemetery. As I was driving through the cemetery, I saw that there was tons and tons of freshly fallen snow everywhere. I looked for footprints as I drove because I wanted to see if anyone had disregarded the cemetery's policy and visited their loved one's grave anyway. There were no footprints. Because I was wearing dress shoes, I thought there was no way I could walk through the snow even if I wanted. I continued to drive and thought, "If only Jesus would make a path for me." It wasn't a prayer, just a thought. As I came upon the section where Sam was buried, the song that I prayed before, during, and after Samuel's death, "Even If" by MercyMe, came on the radio. It's Sam's song, and whenever I hear it, I relive everything and know that Sam is with me in a special way.

For Sam's song to play at that moment was a gift, but it wasn't the only gift. After I parked my car, I started to get out with my daughter Hannah. As I prepared to go toward Sam's grave, I noticed the most unbelievable thing. There was a path. The path started where my car had stopped, continued all the way to where Sam was buried, and ended just a bit beyond. Jesus had plowed a path for me! It was a miracle! Jesus loved me! He knew my pain and made a path so I could be with my son. I cried. When Hannah asked why I was crying, I said, "Jesus made a path for me because He knew I was sad." Hannah asked, "Why are you sad?" I replied, "Today is Sam's due date, and I am sad that he doesn't get the chance to be born." Hannah confidently exclaimed, "Mom, Sam *was* born. *Sam was born into Heaven!*" How did my little girl profess such great wisdom?

My son Sam was born. He was born into Heaven. When a baby is born, everyone rejoices, and they announce the birth and the name of their baby to the world. When someone loses their baby through miscarriage, they never get this opportunity. I am grateful to God for the life of Sam. His life was silent, yet powerful. Sam's life stretched my heart and taught my heart how to love. His life has challenged me not to be indifferent to the sufferings and Passion of Jesus and Mary and not to be indifferent to the sufferings and circumstances of others. His life has given me a new set of eyes, eyes that are more set on Heaven. I am grateful that the Lord chose me to be Sam's mom. If God gave me the choice between experiencing his short life through the agony of miscarriage and not having him at all, I would choose Sam. Sam is alive. He exists. He is in Heaven resting in the arms of Jesus and Mary. Sam is not forgotten or forsaken. Although no one has met, heard, or held our Sam, he has God and a family who love him. Sam will forever be a part of me, forever in my heart, and forever loved, and I cannot wait to begin my forever with Sam in Heaven, where I will hold him forever. As Telly professed the life of her son in the movie *The Forgotten,* today I rejoice and announce the birth of my son, who was born into Heaven. "I had life inside me. I had life. I have a child. I have a son. I... have a son. His name is Sam."

May God be forever praised.

CHAPTER 7

MISCARRIAGE

He Was Only Six Weeks

Jacqui Fetsko

I NEVER THOUGHT I would be writing about baby Michael. Yet, as I look at what God has done for me in my life, this should come as no surprise. I am writing this story for baby Michael. I want to honor him as he should have been honored right from the get-go, twenty years ago. Unknowingly, I had allowed our culture to influence my grieving process. But I digress. The following is my story about our son Michael.

This story begins on a Sunday at church. My husband and I were chatting in the social area when my then nine-year-old daughter, Therese, excitedly ran up to us saying, "I got my rose! I got my rose!" She showed us a chocolate angel that had been given to her, and in the hands of the angel was a chocolate rose. She went on to tell us that she had just finished a novena to St. Thérèse, the Little Flower. She explained that she had been praying for us to have another child! We were very touched by that and thought, "*How sweet.*"

Two weeks later, I found myself pregnant with our fifth child! I will never forget the day when the pregnancy test was positive. You see, I always wanted a large family, at least eight children, and this was such an answer to my prayers. It had been about five and a half years since we had Sarah, our fourth child. After she was born, my husband, Bob, and I decided to use NFP to postpone pregnancy for one year. We had had four children in less than five years, and we thought it would be wise to take a rest. After that year was over, we began to hope for more children and assumed it would be easy, considering the number and ease of our previous pregnancies. How little did we know!

Thus began my desperation to have more children. I would argue with God, asking Him why I was getting my period month after month. I was so angry with Him! (I did confess this anger, by the way.) You see, I thought I *deserved* more children. I was a faithful Catholic, I did not use artificial contraception, I was a pro-life activist and fought hard for the protection of all human life, and I homeschooled my four children. So why was I not getting pregnant? I was told by a priest that God knew my heart and could handle my anger. That did little to comfort me at the time, however. So, when this pregnancy test this time came back positive after so many years, I was beyond happy! I cannot express how joyful I was at the news. I immediately began to plan this baby's life. I would homeschool this little one, and the baby would go to this college, and then … you get the picture.

Providentially, I had a scheduled appointment with the gynecologist for my annual checkup within the week of finding out I was pregnant. On the evening before the appointment, I began some slight spotting. I vaguely remember some dread, but I reminded myself that I had worse spotting with my firstborn, Therese, and she was born in good health.

When I arrived for my appointment the next morning, I let the doctor know about the spotting. He immediately ordered an intrauterine ultrasound. I thank God for this ultrasound, because I was able to see my precious son (not confirmed but instinctually known). There he was in his glory. There was a buildup of the endometrial lining on one side, but there was no sac, as had been hoped for. They attributed that to it being too early for detection or because a miscarriage had already taken place. This was the first and last time I would see my son, or what remained of him.

The doctor ordered blood work to monitor the HCG levels in my blood. The next day, the results showed that the HCG levels were dropping, so miscarriage was imminent. Sure enough, I began to bleed and pass many heavy clots. I distinctly remember sitting on the front sofa, looking out the window, knowing my baby was passing out of me. I have no idea where my husband and children were at the time; I honestly can't recall. I just remember being alone, crying uncontrollably, and feeling overwhelmingly *powerless*. I felt completely out of control, knowing there was nothing I could do to save my child. All my dreams for him were disappearing and leaving me feeling helpless and so very sad.

Three days later, a second intrauterine ultrasound was performed, and there I saw my completely empty womb. He was gone. My baby was no longer with me. Although I knew I had lost him prior to the appointment, the finality of this image of my empty womb was so painful.

What about Therese? How was I to explain to her that her prayer had been answered, even though baby Michael died? Fortunately, God gave me the words to explain that, in fact, she had a brother in Heaven. As children always do, she got it and understood it better than I.

When I was asked to submit this story, I asked Bob how he felt through the miscarriage. He said he was sad but that he was more concerned about me. It was hard on him to see my grief, and he did not know what to do. The children took the news well. They did not struggle with the loss as I did, and they were so young at the time. My son Rob's ninth birthday came two days after our loss. I had informed my family about it, and my parents were sympathetic.

My mom brought a bouquet of yellow daffodils for me during Rob's birthday celebration at our home. My husband's parents said nothing, though. I was terribly hurt by this at the time, but I suspect that they just did not know what to say. (My mother-in-law had also suffered a miscarriage a couple of years after my husband was born.)

As much as I was in turmoil inside, I fought hard to put on a good face. After all, I had four living children, while some couples have none. He was only six weeks along, whereas others have lost children who had been born. My loss did not appear to bother anyone else, so why was I so sad? Millions of unborn children were being butchered by abortion. How could my loss even compare to that? I did not want to offend God by not accepting His will and believed that I just had to move on.

At the time I thought that I was doing well and that I was right in moving on. However, I now realize that I had not permitted myself to grieve as I should have and that I had unknowingly absorbed the culture's ideology regarding the dignity of the unborn. I fell for the lie that grieving for such a young one was not appropriate. After all, he was only six weeks! Years later, a priest and I were discussing an issue related to Christ's humanity, and he pointed out that I was thinking in human terms only. He mentioned that I had unknowingly taken on a worldly view. He was spot on!

I deeply missed Michael. I keep journals and in them I recalled Michael often. I often got sad in December because his due date would have been December 10. My emotions would get a little crazy, and yet I pushed on. In some weird way, I thought I did not deserve to grieve or feel such a heavy loss, and I think this was because I was comparing my loss with others'. Perhaps I was thinking that I would seem ungrateful for all the children I did have. My heart ached, but my outward actions masked the hurt. My sister-in-law had lost four children to miscarriage, one of them reaching seven months gestation. She seemed to move on and keep her joy. Should I not do the same?

As time passed, our family experienced some tragic events. Two close family members had survived attempts at suicide. In one case, the attempt was completely averted because he had been called for just as he was about to follow through. In the second case, the attempt was made, but our family member survived. I believe that Michael interceded in both cases. In fact, he has been a source of strength for me in a particular way. I turn to him in prayer for my other children, especially when they are going through hard times. I know in my heart that he is praying for them and that God grants him his requests.

As I have already said, I did not grieve for Michael as I should have, but in God's tender love for me, He gave me an opportunity to do so. I wish I could remember the date, but I can't. The Catholic parish near my home offers an annual memorial Mass for babies lost through miscarriage, abortion, or any other way. While I am not a parishioner at that church, I attend daily Mass there. I had been aware of this Mass but had not taken the initiative to attend because of my messed-up way of thinking that my loss didn't merit this kind of memorial. This time, for some reason, I decided to go, and I am so glad I did!

I was invited to take a flower and fill out a tag with my baby's name on it. I had not done this apart from my journaling, and once I wrote Michael's name, it was as if I were finally acknowledging the reality of his beautiful life and his inherent value and dignity even at six weeks. It seems so silly that this small action could mean so much to me, but it did. The flowers were placed before the altar in the church, representing the children being remembered that day. After Mass, we were invited to choose a blue or pink balloon. I chose a blue one, and then we attached the tags with our babies' names to the balloons. Then we went outside and released the balloons into the air.

This action was so freeing and so comforting! For the first time I had publicly grieved the loss of Michael.

I recently attended this annual memorial Mass again, and once again wrote Michael's name down and chose a flower to represent him at the altar. His sister Sarah joined me and we also remembered two more babies, baby Natalie and baby Rose, who were my niece's children. Baby Natalie and baby Rose were the first two great-grandchildren on my side of the family.

I still cry over Michael. I regret how I initially handled his loss. I feel guilty that his remains were not buried but were lost among the tissue and blood that passed through me on that day. I regret doubting his reality and wondering whether or not I was imagining his existence. I regret letting the culture cloud my judgment and thinking mostly in human terms. I regret comparing my loss with others. I regret wearing my mask of self-reliance and not being true to my heart, which was so deeply broken. I regret my lack of trust in God, which prevented me from being completely real with Him.

This is my experience, though, and I believe it was for a reason. I do have regrets, but I am not the same person I was when I lost Michael. Losing him was the first step in letting go and letting God be in charge. I did not change overnight, by any stretch of the imagination! It has been a long road, and many failures and extraordinary grace have gotten me to where I am today, with a long road still ahead of me. I can now look back and see God's plan in all of this. He has taught me that life is a gift and not an entitlement. I did not deserve any children, but God granted me five! I did not earn my family; God gave them to me! God does not love me based on what I do, but for who I am — a weak sinner in need of a Savior. I am loved beyond measure in spite of myself. There is absolutely nothing I can do or not do to change that. Losing Michael helped me gain awareness of the abundant love of my Heavenly Father. God took Michael home in order for my family and me to have an intercessor closely linked to us, physically and spiritually. He took Michael and spared him the sufferings of this world. What a gift!

Furthermore, God had a job for me. I would not have been able to do this job had Michael survived. I have been called to deeper pro-life activism and am fulfilling roles I could not have done had I had more children. There have also been family crises that would not have been handled as well if we had more children. I have been able to dedicate my life to these two areas and can see why things worked out the way they did. My family needed Michael in Heaven for us to navigate some of the heavy trials we faced. Without him in Heaven, we would have been lacking the help he provided, as well as the help he continues to give.

Who would have thought that a six-week-old unborn child could have such an impact on my life and the life of my family? I am so extremely grateful to God for Michael. God showed how much He loves me through the gift of Michael, as well as through my husband and four living children. I am so grateful for each and every one of them!

I want to close my story with the journal entry I made on April 16, 1999. I also want to thank Patrick for inviting me to share Michael's and my story. It has been purgative and has enabled me to put into words my journey through loss, grief, lessons learned, and an unwavering trust in my Heavenly Father. Thank you!

> *Before my Lord Jesus Christ in the Blessed Sacrament:*
>
> *I lost my baby today. Oh, I am sad but not completely. I mourned my little one, but God in His goodness has enabled me to carry this cross with some joy, believe it or not. I am grateful for the new life God allowed Bob and I to help create. We know that this baby of ours is in Heaven, praying for his parents and siblings. The children and I have named him Michael.*

Michael, I hope God has let you know how much you are loved by your family. We only knew of you for a week and a half, but you had given us such happiness, and through you, God instilled hope — the hope that more children may be granted to our family, which longs for more! Michael, I am suffering over the loss of you in my earthly life, but through you, God enables me to embrace His will for me. Through you, dear Michael, I have learned that I lacked trust in God the Father, and I am so sorry for that. Once I placed my all in His hands, He comforted me — and I owe this to you, dear Michael. Michael, pray for me, your father, and your siblings. Intercede for us so that we completely place our lives in our Heavenly Father's hands. I kiss you with my heart and wash you with my tears, dear little one. I will never forget you.

CHAPTER 8

Miscarriage

Our First Baby

Peter McClone

I HATE SHOPPING. I have always hated shopping, especially for clothes. But this shopping trip was fun. We went from store to store in the Anne Arundel Mall, looking at the tiniest baby clothes and the accessories — bibs, socks, and all the rest. We did not end up buying much, but it was so exciting just looking and thinking about our new baby. Would we have a boy or a girl? What was it going to be like to be parents?

What made it even more fun was that we were not alone. My parents had flown in, and we were able to share the amazing news with them. Ruth was pregnant! My grandma was there, too. We wheeled her around the mall in a borrowed wheelchair, and she insisted that *she* buy the outfits. This was going to be her first great-grandchild and she was excited too.

The bottom line is that Ruth and I could not have been happier. We had been married for about six months and had been trying to have a baby since our wedding day. Although we knew we had a lot to learn and there was a lot to do, honestly, there was not a worry on my mind. We didn't wait very long to tell people and start getting prepared.

I didn't really know how pregnancy worked. I didn't know how frequently Ruth needed to go to the doctor, if she should be eating differently, or if there was anything else we should do. This is why I was really excited when we got an offer to have a free early ultrasound. *Everything* was exciting.

There was a pro-life clinic in the area that had just received an ultrasound machine, and they were training their staff to use it. When we were there for a fundraiser one weekend, the staff offered to give us an ultrasound as part of the training. How cool was that!

I was not prepared at all for what this meant. I do not remember what day of the week it was or even the time of day. I remember it was sunny and warm. We went in, sat down, and waited. I had never seen an ultrasound before. I didn't know what to expect, and I didn't know what I would see.

The nurse welcomed us. She congratulated us and helped Ruth get on the bed. Once she got on there, my eyes were *fixed* on the screen. We held hands.

If you have never seen an ultrasound, they always start out as blobs. It was a mess of black-and-white pixels flying across the screen. The nurse moved the wand around and we just watched the blobs. I was excited and was trying to make out what I was looking at.

She moved the wand around some more. I started to watch the nurse to try to get a clue as to what I should be looking at on the screen. This is when I noticed a change in her demeanor. It became serious, and she looked at the other staff member in the room. I didn't know what to say or to ask. She kept moving the wand, so I just kept watching and waiting. I felt Ruth's grip tighten. We were both wondering, "*What is going on?*"

After a few more minutes, I heard, "I'm sorry." That's all she said. "*What does that mean — I'm sorry?*" I said to myself. I looked at Ruth. We were both so confused. I think the nurse said something about what we should say to Ruth's doctor. I really don't know what happened next. All I remember is holding Ruth in my arms in the sunny, warm parking lot while she cried. I held her for a long time.

Over the next few days we found out more. It turns out that our baby had died. Another ultrasound confirmed that the baby had stopped growing at about six weeks.

We prayed so hard. Over those few days that was all we could do. We prayed and cried. We prayed that a miracle would occur and the baby would come back to life. We asked God why this happened. We asked Him to take the pain away. We begged Our Lady to be with us. I have never prayed so hard in my life.

In our confusion and pain, we reached out to a lot of family and friends. The response was overwhelming. There was so much support and prayer that surrounded us. Ruth's doctor recommended a D&C, which is a surgery that would remove the baby and other tissue to help Ruth heal physically. Emotionally, we were so distraught. We thought, *"If only we pray hard enough, God will miraculously bring this baby back to life."*

After so much prayer, we consulted a friend from college who was a nurse experienced in this area. She helped us understand that following the advice of our doctor was probably the best course of action. We will always be eternally grateful for the phone calls and prayers from her.

While Ruth's doctor may have been an expert in medicine, he certainly was not in charity. When we went in to talk to him about the surgery and schedule it, we nervously asked for the remains of our baby to take home afterward. "Why?" he asked bluntly. "Don't you know how big it is? It's this big!" he said, holding two fingers close together. We were in so much pain, and he either couldn't see it or didn't care. Like many people then (and later), he simply thought that we wanted a child and didn't get one. But we knew we had a child and lost it.

The surgery day was long, but it was a prayerful day. In a way it brought some closure to the event. Again, a generous and holy friend all the way across the country was key to making the day bearable. Knowing what was going on, that friend promised to pray throughout the day for us. Sometimes you can just feel prayers, and I did that day.

The surgery went well. Afterward, the nurses gave us the remains of our baby. We went home and slept. I do not think we had really been able to sleep until that day. I would never wish this suffering on anyone, but it is amazing how it produces opportunities for love. There was a wonderful old priest at Holy Trinity in Glen Burnie, Maryland. I had been going to morning Mass there as much as possible for a year or so. Father graciously offered to have Mass and a service for us.

The pastor of our parish, Our Lady of the Fields, was also kind. He offered to hold a burial service and gave us a spot to bury the remains in the parish cemetery. "*Do you buy a headstone for an unborn child?*" I wondered. I did not know what to do, so we buried him with a parishioner who had recently passed.

We invited a few friends to the burial, but we did not really expect them to come. But they did come. We had five good friends there. Brendan, a friend from Bible study, showed up dressed in a full suit. He gave me a huge hug that I will never forget. Real friends share your pain as well as your joys.

After weeks of intense prayer and emotion, I started to recover a bit. (Ruth took a lot longer.) But we both became drawn to a particular image of Our Lady in our parish that we had never noticed before. It looked very familiar. We asked if it was new and were told that it had been there since the church was built.

While we tried to go to daily Mass frequently before the miscarriage, we were driven to go every day after. We would drive thirty miles to find a Mass we could make work each day. We discovered that the "familiar" image was so familiar because it was prominently displayed in *every church* we went to. It was the image of Our Lady of Perpetual Help.

We had been praying and praying, and Our Lady's response was, "I will be your perpetual help!" As I mentioned, Ruth took a long time to heal emotionally. Losing Pete Jr. was not something to "get over," but we did learn to be grateful for the gift of his life.

Eventually, through Natural Family Planning and the help of a great Catholic doctor, we discovered that Ruth has a progesterone deficiency. Although we did suffer another miscarriage, whom we named Gerard, we have also been blessed with five beautiful, healthy children. We have also shared prayers, pain, and hope with many other couples who have suffered miscarriage.

Our lives are different because of each one of our children. God has stretched our hearts and helped deepen our love for Him and for each other. We hope that in reading this story, God will change your heart too.

Our Lady of Perpetual Help, pray for us!

CHAPTER 9

Miscarriage

Ada Marie's Story

Lyndsey Day

"For this I was born, and for this I have come into the world, to bear witness to the truth" (John 18:37).

As an ob-gyn, I am so lucky to get to walk with women on some of the best days of their lives. I read once that the veil between Heaven and earth is thin at the time of birth. Maybe that is why I cherish deliveries so much — being close to our Creator in those miraculous moments when a brand-new life enters this world for the first time. Those first breaths. There is no joy quite as deep as that of a mother holding her long-awaited child for the first time. It is an honor to be one of the lucky few who gets to stand in that moment, who gets to walk with women into and through motherhood.

But I also walk with women on some of the worst days of their lives — days when unfortunately the veil between Heaven and earth is not thin enough, when that baby is just beyond reach. There is no sorrow quite as deep as that of a mother who has just learned that she will forever walk this earth with a piece of her heart missing. It is an honor to share in those moments, too, and I remember the women who walk away empty. I remember your babies. I know their names.

They will always be a part of my story, a part of my heart. But I never thought my story would involve my own loss. I never thought my baby's name would be etched on the heart of my doctors. I walk with women through their grief. I was not expecting my own.

When we found out we were expecting our fifth baby, I was a little shocked and a little nervous. Five kids seemed like a lot. But my apprehensions quickly faded, and we began to prepare for what life would be like with a new baby in our family. We soon learned our baby was a girl, and the early screenings we did were normal. She was perfect and healthy, and we could breathe a sigh of relief. We decided that my husband could name this one, but I wanted to be surprised. I wanted him to tell me her name when they placed her on my chest in the delivery room. We could not wait to meet her.

One of the many blessings of being an ob-gyn is ready access to an ultrasound machine and a dear friend to scan me. So, one night after work, I wanted to take a quick look and check on our girl. In those moments, my life changed forever. Instantly, we could both see something was wrong. The scenarios that I had walked through with other women were now right before me. My head was spinning and my heart was breaking, but I tried to hope for the best. We could manage a baby with a special medical condition. We would be fine with a child with special needs. I prayed that we would be able to bring this baby home. I could not imagine how I would survive any other outcome.

Somehow, we walked through the next few days until I was able to get an ultrasound at the University of Iowa. That day, the Gospel reading was the one in which Jesus healed the ten lepers (Luke 17:11–19). I reflected on this reading as we drove an hour to see a specialist for our appointment. Radical healing. Miraculous healing! Was this what the Lord had in store for us? I was struck by the Samaritan who returned to Jesus after being healed, the only one out of the ten. Can you imagine that moment? For that man to be completely healed and fall at the feet of Jesus in praise and thanksgiving! I read a devotion that day that said, "Maybe the Gospel writers shared this story with the Church, not only to show us the incredible saving power of Christ, but to allow us to encounter healing as a simple returning to the Source of all life. The complexities of fear and doubt have no power over the One who brings us back to total restoration. There is no striving, earning, or posturing. At the feet of the Messiah, there is healing and returning."

Healing as a simple returning to the Source of all life. At the feet of the Messiah there is healing and returning. I did not like the sound of this. This felt like a sign that my baby would be returning to God before I wanted her to, returning to the Source of life to be completely healed. This felt like God trying to prepare my heart for something I did not want. I fell at His feet.

On the drive to the ultrasound appointment, I wrote in my journal, "Either we will find out that you are fine and healthy and we have nothing to fear, or we may find out that our life with you might look different than we thought. While I pray that we find out nothing is wrong, I know that this might not be God's plan for you. I will trust Him and His plan for I know it is good. How shortsighted I would be if I thought my plan was better than the plan of our God, who works in eternity. You are so loved. So many are praying for you. There is no way this can go wrong. We are protected, surrounded, and loved. I love you so much. I am honored to be your mom. I am thankful for however long I get to love you here physically with me and I pray that it is for all of my days."

The moment the ultrasonographer began scanning, I started to panic. I could not believe this was happening. I could very clearly see that my baby's spine was curved like a *J*, there was no separation between her abdomen and the placenta, and all of her organs seemed to be growing outside her abdomen. Her legs were twisted to the side and behind her. Something was very wrong. We were not going to get to bring her home. I wondered if my husband could tell by the images. I couldn't breathe. I couldn't tell him. A kind doctor came in and confirmed what I already knew. "Limb body wall complex" is what our daughter had. No chance of survival after birth. A fatal condition. Our daughter would not live. Yet I just saw her kicking and moving her hands, and her heart was beating. How could this be? I asked my husband for her name — Ada Marie. Her name means "adorned." It was the perfect name. My strong and wonderful husband held me and somehow we made our way out of the hospital. We got in our car, with pictures of our sweet, perfect girl, and headed home.

I cannot begin to describe what the next few days were like. We were devastated. We were in disbelief. Could this be a mistake? How will we survive this? Will our kids really have to go to their sister's funeral? We begged God to take this away, to heal our baby. We prayed on our knees. We asked everyone we knew to pray, and the outpouring of love and support was overwhelming. People from all over the world, people we had never met, people from different faiths and situations, were all united in hope and love and prayer for our Ada Marie. We would keep Ada with us as long as God intended. God has always provided for us, so we asked Him to lead us gently.

"Rejoice in your hope, be patient in tribulation, be constant in prayer" (Rom. 12:12). As we walked through those days, we spent time oscillating between hope, despair, and complete love and gratitude that we had been given the gift of sweet Ada Marie. Receiving the diagnosis that your baby has a fatal condition is like walking through a bunch of traumatic events over and over again. It isn't just one hard blow. It is the diagnosis that maybe something is wrong. Then a little hope that maybe it is not. Then making some new plans and doing a lot of research and holding on to hope. Then the blow that yes, indeed, something is very wrong, and then, still, a little hope. Maybe someone can fix this? Maybe we just need to find the right doctor? Maybe they are wrong. Maybe there will be a miracle. Then facing the facts that they are right and there is no doctor who can fix this. Our hopes changed — some days we hoped and prayed for miraculous healing, others we hoped for time with Ada. We hoped to hear her cry or to see her eyes or to hold her in our arms when she died. We made more new plans. We carried her with us and loved her as much as we could.

I have always had a very strong devotion to Mary. As a woman and a mother, I try to walk close to her and follow her example of faith. She said yes to something very scary. She endured much suffering. But she trusted the Lord always. The Annunciation, her *fiat,* is something I felt very close to through my pregnancy with Ada. Before us was something very scary. Before us was much suffering. So, like Mary, we too sought to trust in the Lord and said, "May it be done according to your word." An excerpt from the chapter "Mothers of God" in the book *Gospel Medicine* really spoke to me during this time:

> In thinking of the annunciation, of Mary's fiat — she had a choice — whether to say yes to it or no, whether to take hold of the unknown life the angel held out to her or whether to defend herself against it however she could.
>
> Terrible things happen and wonderful things happen, but seldom do we know ahead of time what will happen to us. Like Mary, our choices often boil down to yes or no. Yes I will live this life that is being held out to me or no, I will not. Yes I will explore this unexpected turn of events or no, I will not. If you decide no, you simply drop your eyes and refuse to look up again until you know the angel has left the room. You go back to your life and pretend that nothing happened. If your life begins to change you can

> be stoic. You can refuse to accept it. You can put all of your energy into ignoring it and insist in spite of everything that it is not happening to you. If that doesn't work, you become angry, actively defending yourself against the unknown and spending all of your time trying to get your life back the way it used to be. And then you become bitter, comparing yourself to everyone else whose lives are more agreeable than yours and lamenting your unhappy life. If you succeed, your life may not be an easy one, but you can rest assured that no angels will trouble you again.
>
> Or you can say yes. You can decide to be a daredevil and listen to the strange creature's plan. You can decide to take part in a plan you did not choose. You can agree to smuggle God into the world inside your own body. Deciding to say yes does not mean you are not afraid. So you say yes to the angel. You say "here I am, let it be done to me according to your word" and you become one who is willing to bear God into the world.[32]

Some days, the despair was overwhelming. But there were also moments of overwhelming beauty and love. We had many moments when we just loved her. We talked to her. We listened to her heartbeat. The kids told her about ice cream and snow days and Christmas. They patted my stomach and told her they loved her. It was a time when our hearts were stretched so much that they were completely shattered at both the sorrow and the beauty of love. We planned her funeral while praying for a miracle. We planned for her delivery. We planned what music we wanted her to hear, what blankets we wanted her to feel on her skin, who would meet her. We planned for a

[32] Barbara Brown Taylor, *Gospel Medicine* (Cambridge, MA: Cowley Publications, 1995), 164–168.

Baptism in the hospital, for many pictures and videos to be taken. We prayed for an easy delivery that wouldn't be too traumatic for her little body. We prayed she would not have any pain and we planned palliative care for her. We prayed for lots of time with her and that we would be holding her when she went to Heaven. We prayed that we would get to hear her cry and see her eyes and kiss her cheeks and feel the weight of her in our arms and on our chests. We prayed for the grace to survive all of this.

"May those who sow in tears reap with shouts of joy! He that goes forth weeping, bearing the seed of sowing, shall come home with shouts of joy, bringing his sheaves with him" (Ps. 126:5–6). On December 5, we went in for an ultrasound, just so we could see her and spend some time with her. She was so very beautiful! She was sucking her thumb, swallowing, moving, kicking! She looked so strong and so very good. We were so fortunate to get many pictures and videos of her. Her heartbeat was perfect and we thought that maybe her defects were not as bad as we had initially thought. Her umbilical cord appeared to have grown — something we had prayed for! Maybe God really did have a miracle in store for our girl! I read article after article, medical and radiology journals, accounts of miracles. I petitioned many saints. I searched through Scripture. I sent prayer requests that traveled around the country. We had hope. The next day, I felt Ada move for the first time.

On Sunday night, December 9, the most wonderful people held the most beautiful prayer service for our Ada Marie. The church was completely full. Full of our dearest family and friends. Full of people we didn't know. Full of *love*. Full of people who loved Ada and prayed for her and believed that the God of the universe had created Ada for a reason that was good and that His plan is perfect. It was a miraculous night. There were beautiful Scripture readings, prayers, and songs. So many hearts were united in love. I wish that everyone could have a moment like this in their lives. It was a night of life and love and celebration of the gift of a child — the one I was carrying, and the one we were preparing our hearts for on that second Sunday of Advent. We left the church that night with hearts full. We were filled with peace. God was leading us gently and His provision was abundant.

The next day, with hearts still overflowing, I sensed a change. I didn't feel Ada anymore. I tried to shake off the feeling. She was still little, and she had looked so good a few days before on the ultrasound. We had an appointment scheduled the following week, and I figured we could wait until then to get checked out. But Tuesday brought more uneasiness, and by Wednesday, I needed to check on her.

God met me there, in that ultrasound room. But Ada did not. I looked at my baby, but she was gone at eighteen weeks. The screen was still. Where a few days ago had been a strong and bouncing baby was now a tiny girl, curled into a little ball, with a heart that had stopped beating. We did not have enough time with her! We were supposed to get to hold her when she died! Why did she leave like this? We realized that she must have died at the prayer service on Sunday night. It was her calling home. It was her send-off to Heaven. In fact, God did have a miracle in store for Ada. It was just not the way we pictured it. She was lifted to Our Lord with so many voices in prayer and song and praise! A baby, born into the arms of Jesus, only knowing love in her life.

The stillness on the ultrasound screen was then followed by even more things that we did not want to face. The delivery, the handprints, the saying goodbye, the going home empty, and the walking through the rest of our lives on earth without a piece of our hearts. How would we ever smile again? None of it was how this was supposed to go. It was not the way we thought Ada would enter the world, but I guess she wasn't really intended for that anyway. "For we do not want you to be ignorant, brethren, of the affliction we experienced in Asia; for we were so utterly, unbearably crushed that we despaired of life itself. Why, we felt that we had received the sentence of death; but that was to make us rely not on ourselves but on God who raises the dead" (2 Cor. 1:8–9).

So we began our dance of sorrow and joy. It really is not much of a dance, though. The waves of grief are overpowering and knock me down again just when I start to get back up. I am in awe of how a mother's story and the story of her child are so intricately woven together. I was chosen for Ada, just as much as she was chosen for me. It is such a weird thing to feel — that Ada was just … gone. Here one minute, gone the next. I still can't really wrap my mind around it. I am still waiting for a sign from her. I just want to see her, to feel her once more. I want a dream or a sign or something! I keep searching for her every day.

But I was praying the Rosary shortly after Ada died, my favorite joyful mysteries, and I caught my breath as I meditated on the fifth joyful mystery — the Finding of Jesus in the Temple. Mary was frantic. Searching for her son — oh, her poor heart! I know exactly how she must have felt, looking everywhere for her beloved boy; she must have been so scared. And then to finally find him in the Temple, and he said to her, "Mother why did you search for me? Didn't know you I would be in the house of my father?" Oh, sweet Jesus. Oh, sweet Mary. Oh, sweet Ada. Of course. Why am I so frantically looking for you here? I know where you are.

In Romans 8:15–18, we hear the words: "For you did not receive the spirit of slavery to fall back into fear, but you have received the spirit of sonship. When we cry, 'Abba! Father!' it is the Spirit himself bearing witness with our spirit that we are children of God, and if children, then heirs, heirs of God and fellow heirs with Christ, provided we suffer with him in order that we may also be glorified with him." If we suffer with Jesus, we will be glorified with Him. Our present sufferings are not worth comparing to the glory that is coming.

Following the loss of Ada, we decided to study the book of Job during Lent. We bought a family study called "Suffering and the God Who Speaks" and clawed our way through it together. I never would have read the book of Job if it were not for our circumstances at the time. It is *tough* to read. A good and righteous and faithful man loses everything, including his ten children, his property, his wealth, his health. But the thing about this is, the devil had to ask God's permission to tempt Job. God is not the author of this evil. He does not cause bad things to happen. However, He did pick Job because he knew that Job would carry the suffering well. Job would suffer well. Because suffering can also point to God's glory.

Job's suffering was an honor, a privilege. "Shall we receive good at the hand of God, and shall we not receive evil?" (Job 2:10). It was an honor for Job to carry the weight of pain. Divine suffering. And I was given a new lens to view some of my suffering through: to think of this as a journey that God handpicked us to take, knowing that He would provide us with all that we needed for the journey and, more importantly, that God's glory would be illuminated through us.

This also made me think about another man who was handpicked to share in suffering—Simon of Cyrene. A man just going about his business one minute and forced to help Jesus carry the Cross to Golgotha the next. How horrible that must have been! Simon did not want to help Jesus carry the Cross. He was not volunteering to help Jesus. I am sure he would have done anything to get out of it. But I think about now, if we saw Jesus Christ walking down our street carrying His Cross, how so many would run to Him, would absolutely take the Cross from Him! There would be many fighting at a chance to carry the Cross of Jesus, to be that close to Him, even to touch his Cross. Divine suffering. An honor to carry the weight of pain.

I was sitting in Adoration on a peaceful night in February. I felt like I had not moved much at all in nearly three months since I last had Ada with me. Three months. A quarter of a year. How much had changed? How much was still the same? In three months, I felt my grief was just as strong, my sorrow just as painful, my loss just as big. I felt like I was right where I started. And maybe that is because I was. I was not actually walking anywhere. I was actually sitting at the foot of the Cross. And that is an okay place to be, sitting before Our Lord in His suffering and sorrow, next to His mother in her heartbreak. It was an excruciating journey to get there. It is awful and lonely and heartbreaking to be there. But yet, I was there in good company — before my Lord and next to His mother. What an incredible honor to share in this Cross, in this moment with them! To share our sorrow, to share our love. There is such beauty and glory at the foot of the Cross. *So much love*! So I decided to just keep sitting there as long as God wanted me to. Until He wanted me to go to the tomb. He is good while I sit at the foot of the Cross. He has never left me. He is before me in complete love. Even in the darkness, before the next good thing happens. What is true in the light is still true in the dark.

“So you have sorrow now, but I will see you again and your hearts will rejoice, and no one will take your joy from you” (John 16:22).

I do not believe that God causes heartache or awful things to happen. But He is with us in our suffering, and He will use it for good if we let Him. But I do not want it to be forgotten that God is not only good in that empty tomb in the light of Easter morning, He is also so very good right now. He is good in the waiting. He is good in the sorrow. He is good in the dark. He is working all things for good, and just because I might not see it or know how it will be, I will not be shortsighted enough to ignore that there is truly nothing too marvelous for our God, the God of the universe. And so I will wait. I will surrender. I will trust. For I know nothing can compare to the glory that will be revealed through the story of my sweet Ada Marie.

CHAPTER 10

Miscarriage

George's Story

Nicole Swannack

It had been seven years since giving birth to my youngest child. Seven years of expecting a sixth pregnancy that never came. Seven years of longing for the blessing of another child. Then, in December 2022, there I stood with a positive pregnancy test in hand. Incomprehensible joy and gratitude overwhelmed me as I stared at the two pink lines on the test. I photographed the test and texted it to my husband, who was away on travel, to make sure it was real.

My husband confirmed the presence of these pink lines and probably wondered why I needed his confirmation. After having five children, I could surely read a pregnancy test myself, but sometimes, when the thing that you so desire is given to you, you need someone else to pinch you to know that you're not dreaming.

I praised God that morning as I attended Mass, thanking Him for this child and the incredible blessing of new life. During prayer, the name George was given to me for the new baby. So, George it was! The baby had a name and I began to plan. What would life be like when George arrived? I could feel the love and warmth my other children would shower upon him. I mentally rearranged the rooms in our house so that there would be room for him to sleep.

I even anticipated the reaction of my fifteen- and sixteen-year-old girls when they were told they would have to return to sharing a room to accommodate the new baby (which made me laugh).

I experienced all of the excitement, beauty, and love that accompany the news of pregnancy. In a small way, I imagine that these are the sentiments Our Lord has as He loves us into being, planning the good works we shall do in Christ Jesus. "For we are his workmanship, created in Christ Jesus for good works, which God prepared beforehand, that we should walk in them" (Eph. 2:10).

All was well until the feast of the Baptism of Our Lord. On this day, I miscarried George. There are no words to express the sorrow I felt over his loss. There was a deep ache within me. Confusion and doubt rooted. Why would my good and loving Lord bless me with a child, only to take him away? What could be the purpose of a life so short? These two questions consumed my mind and eventually sowed doubt over the value of such a young life. Was George actually a beloved son of God, or was that simply wishful thinking? Maybe he was actually just a clump of cells after all? Could someone so small, so young, be in Heaven with our Father? Did God really create George, know George, love George?

My husband and I told our five children that we had lost the pregnancy. I cried, I prayed, and then I packed up my feelings, pushed aside my doubts, and moved on. The world doesn't stop because of the pain of some, and so, willingly or begrudgingly, we must carry on. My family and I didn't share the joyous news of our pregnancy or the heartbreaking news of our miscarriage with anyone. We held these events in our hearts, surrendering them to God while also questioning Him.

Weeks passed and the status quo in our family prevailed. I continued praying and attending daily Mass. I taught our parish children,

I taught my own children, I spoke of the love of God, and all the while, a giant thornbush of doubt was growing inside of me. I didn't doubt the existence of God. I didn't even doubt my love for God. Over the weeks I was able to surrender the events to His holy will. However, there was a question that nagged me constantly. Where was my baby?

I began seeing advertisements for a healing service at a local parish, St. Michael's Catholic Church, hosted by the Encounter School. I felt a very strong call to attend this Mass. I convinced myself that I should at least try to seek healing for my fifteen-year-old daughter, who was born with epilepsy, and for my sixteen-year old-daughter, who was plagued by constant anxiety. I didn't really know if I believed that healing services could have an impact on our lives, but I wasn't willing to commit to their futility either. I just didn't know what to think, so it was better to play it safe and give the healing service a shot. What's the worst that could happen? So, I informed my family that we were spending our Friday night at St. Michael's, and off we went.

To my surprise, my children were excited about the evening and were genuinely curious about what this would entail. They approached it with the faith of children, innocent and trusting. Only a short while into the evening my ten-year-old daughter, Rose, declared to us that her broken pinky finger had been completely healed by Jesus. She asked us if she could go to the microphone and give her testimony. We allowed her to do this, not thinking much of it, and not really sure what to think.

For the second half of the evening, the congregation was given the opportunity to wait in line for individual healing. My daughters and I got in line to pray with Fr. Gonyeau and we waited, and waited, and waited.

The wait was extensive but peaceful. It was an opportunity to witness others being prayed over and being healed by Jesus. The presence of the Holy Spirit was palpable and stirred excitement and anticipation within me and my daughters. At some point during our wait, a prayer team of two women approached my family. These women, whom I had never met before, stated that they felt that the Holy Spirit was directing them to come over to our area of the line and pray with someone in the vicinity. I behaved as a dutiful mother and pushed my epileptic daughter toward them, asking them to pray for her. These women prayed over my fifteen-year-old daughter, but declared that she was not the one they were sent to pray for.

"Who else could we pray for?" was their question.

If not for Bridget, then they must need to pray for my Charlotte. Once again, I presented them with a daughter. Prodding my oldest forward, I introduced her and declared that she must be the one they needed to pray for. Maybe the Holy Spirit told them to pray for Charlotte?

Maybe they were just wandering around the parish and this was all nonsense? Either way, their prayers couldn't do any harm.

The women prayed over Charlotte, and then they said, "We need to pray over you."

I assured them that I did not need prayers or healing. I had nothing to be healed of. That said, if they wanted to pray for me, then sure, why not? I didn't want to offend these women, and they were clearly incredibly well intentioned. They did just spend time praying for both of my daughters. So, I resigned to be prayed over. I smiled and hoped that my uncertainty about all of this wasn't written all over my face.

The women started praying and said that they got a message that I had a strong devotion to Our Lady. They were correct. I do have a strong devotion to Mary. "*Okay,*" I thought. "*We are in a Catholic Church, standing here at ten o'clock at night. I'm sure everyone here has a devotion to Mary.*"

They went on to tell me that I've clung to Mary since childhood. And again, they were correct. However, this was yet another thing that could probably have been said for many attending the service.

The feeling that this whole prayer session was silly and nonsensical was welling up within me, and yet there was a part of me that clung to the belief that we were there for a reason.

What happened next changed everything. One of the women said that she saw Mary standing in front of me holding a baby. The woman said that she didn't know who the baby was, because this baby was not Jesus. Upon hearing those words I knew exactly who this baby was.

This baby was George, and Mary had brought him to me.

Tears began streaming down my face as I weakly said that I had miscarried in January. The woman then asked, "Do you want to know the baby's gender?"

I already knew the baby's gender. His name had been given to me in prayer. I didn't share this information with the prayer team. Would these women confirm the words that I had received in prayer, that this was a little baby boy? I waited. God knew that this was the last confirmation I needed to restore my faith.

"The baby is a boy. Mary is caring for him."

This statement confirmed everything and immediately I was revived. All doubt was cast out. My faith rose up like a flame and I blurted out, "Yes, we named him George."

God loves my child. He was intentionally loved into being. He is with the Father in Heaven. He is being cared for by the greatest mother, Mary. And God has a plan for George and for me.

I was told other things that evening by this prayer team. There were prophetic words for the fruit that would be born from this suffering. Words that God would pour forth healing and love on mothers, fathers, and families through George's story.

Most importantly, though, God restored my faith through the prophetic words that came from these two beautiful people. I no longer doubt. I can say with confidence that each child is precious to God and to Mary. We are loved and known before we are formed in our mother's wombs. Our merciful and loving God has a purpose for each of us, regardless of the length of our earthly life.

I left that night desiring a deeper relationship with God. I didn't know how these women could have supernatural encounters. I didn't understand what prophetic words were. All I knew is that I wanted what they had. I wanted more God, more Holy Spirit. I desired this not just for myself, but for my family, my friends, and my students. I desire it for everyone.

About a week after the healing service, I was at Mother Teresa Parish. It was a Saturday evening in February when our parish priest, Fr. Daniel, told me to stop by his office. He had left a present for me on his desk that he wanted me to grab. It was completely out of character for him to give me a present for no reason, so I was very curious. I walked to my car, sat down, and opened the present. I was in complete disbelief when I unwrapped his present. Father had given me a beautiful icon of St. George that he had bought at an antique shop years ago. Fr. Dan had absolutely no knowledge of my pregnancy, miscarriage, or the events that transpired at the healing service. I still hadn't spoken of the miscarriage or the events of the healing service with anyone other than my immediate family. I didn't want people to think I was strange or a crazy Catholic, so I kept all of these things to myself.

I went to him the moment I saw what he had given me and asked, "Did you know?" I knew his answer before he spoke. "Know what?"

"Why did you give this to me?" I asked. He explained that he was going through his possessions and thought that he should give this to me and my family. He was inspired to give this to us, and that is what he did.

Truly, this icon was a gift from the Holy Spirit Himself. Knowing how prone I am to doubt, God gave me a visual reminder that George was in Heaven. Whenever lies or doubt want to creep into my thoughts, I only need to pray before St. George's icon and be reminded of God's love and faithfulness. This gift emboldened me with the courage to share George's story for the greater glory of God.

While healing occurred and my faith was restored, there remained one question lingering in my mind and prayer: Why did my child die? Wouldn't the world have been better off with George in it? Our good and generous Lord answered this question on All Saints' Day that same year. George had been on my mind during that All Saints' Day Mass, and after receiving Holy Communion, I sang and knelt in prayer. The presence of the Lord was palpable, and despite the movement of those around me, I became engulfed in a holy stillness. It was in this divine silence that the voice of God could be heard. "George is home. He is with my mother, his heavenly mother. He is fulfilling his purpose."

The Lord then allowed me to have a brief glimpse of George, and in this moment, he was no longer a baby but a young man. Though his appearance was more mature, he was fully and undoubtedly George, my child. This radiant young man was powerfully praying, interceding, and actively loving from Heaven. Mary was by his side with her peaceful smile, the smile of a mother gazing upon her beloved child. The Father's love radiated from both Mary and George and penetrated me, leaving me convinced of the immense love that the saints and Our Lady have for us. Before George and Mary left, I was permitted to see several people that he was interceding for both on earth and in Purgatory. The impact that these intercessory prayers had on the conversion of earthly souls was incredible. May we beg God for the grace to never underestimate prayer and to never neglect our prayer life! I asked George and Mary to continue to pray for me, my husband, and our living children. I asked them to pray for family, friends, and acquaintances, both living and deceased.

And then I was asked something. Was I willing to accept that this was George's purpose? Yes.

From the moment God blessed me with children, making me a mother, my sole aim has been to raise saints who glorify God with lives of love and service, leading others to Christ. As I've watched my five living children grow and develop, it has become clear that God will work through each of them uniquely, directing and guiding them so that they may be sanctified and so that others may be sanctified by Him through them. My heavenly child, George, is no different than my earthly children. George lives his purpose in Heaven, glorifying God through prayer, through intercession, and through drawing those of us still on earth ever closer to Christ. Each of us is God's masterpiece, created in Christ Jesus with a purpose.

The Lord's kindness and love have healed and strengthened me. George's intercession, along with the intercession of our Blessed Mother and countless other saints, leads all of us closer to Christ each day.

CHAPTER 11

Miscarriage

When the Lord Taketh Away

Kristin Giganti

God has blessed my husband and me with five beautiful children here on this earth. They are our most abundant and treasured blessing. The Lord giveth so generously to us! This is the reality that those around us can see. What many people don't realize is that we are actually parents to eight children.

Sadly, we have lost three tiny babies to miscarriage over the years. In November 2004, about eleven months after our first son was born, our second baby, whom we named Angela Michelle, was lost to miscarriage at approximately six weeks gestation. We were stunned and saddened. The busyness of caring for our young son helped to ease the grieving process, but the experience was one we knew would leave us permanently changed. We lovingly referred to "your little sister Angela" often — and still do, in an effort to keep the memory of her short life a part of ours.

Four beautiful babies and eleven years later, we were blindsided. Life with our four sons and one daughter was typical, and miscarriage was the last thing on our minds. I really did not think it would ever happen again. I had five healthy children. "*My first miscarriage must have been a tragic exception,"* I thought. Yet at almost ten weeks pregnant, we were told our baby had no heartbeat.

The news was delivered by a doctor I had never met, who was detached and medical and likely considered herself extremely professional. As I was slightly past the point where most miscarriages progress naturally, the doctor offered me the choice to "speed things along" by having the surgical procedure known as a D&C. While not necessarily opposed to such an option, I inquired about the possibility of miscarrying outside of a hospital setting. "*Was this safe?*" I wondered.

It is stunning how very little women are told about the reality of miscarriage — either the medical facts or the emotional and physical toll. There is no "industry standard." This is slowly changing, but we have far to go. At this point, I felt wholly unsure of what to expect. I knew instinctively that, physically, a miscarriage at ten weeks was something very different than one at six weeks. But the doctor assured me that I could go home and "let nature take its course," and I would be fine. I thought maybe she would give me a pamphlet or printouts — instructions of some kind. Unfortunately, I was sent on my way with nothing more than a sympathetic smile.

My miscarriage at ten weeks was nothing like my miscarriage at six weeks. Were it not for the loving yet practical advice I received from a wonderful friend who had endured the same tragedy only weeks earlier, I would have been consumed with anxiety about what to expect.

While some women safely miscarry in their own home, my experience was to be more complicated. Traumatic, actually. Less than a week after I sat in the doctor's office, the physical miscarriage process began. For approximately four hours, I was huddled in my bathroom, assuming this was how things were supposed to go. Tragically, the doctor who assured me the process was safe to go through at home neglected to inform me of the risks or what a miscarriage gone wrong looks like. Thus I did not realize that after four hours I was going into shock from blood loss — until I collapsed onto the bathroom floor, barely conscious. By the grace of God, I mustered every ounce of my strength to use my cell phone to call downstairs to my husband: "I need an ambulance, fast."

Our five children watched in tears as EMTs carried me out the front door of our home. I feared I would bleed to death in the time it took to prep for surgery. But in our weakest moments, God is our strength. Even though we lost our seventh child that day, we held to the faith that "God's ways are not our ways."

Even with the aid of our faith, the grief — compounded by the trauma of a life-threatening emergency and subsequent recovery — was profound. I was keenly aware that the world outside kept marching along, while I just needed life to take a pause so I could process things and maybe eventually catch up. I think what I wanted most at that time was time itself; just to carve out a small window to mourn and get myself together.

But time waits for no one, as they say. After a quiet memorial service, we were able to bury our baby, Xavier Paul, in a special section of a local cemetery reserved for infants — at no cost, save discounted funeral home services and an optional gravestone. It was then that I made the horrifying discovery that not all parents are allowed to bury the tiny remains of their children. As I shared with fellow mothers the wonderful program offered by our local Catholic hospital system, whereby infant remains are provided a permanent resting place, I heard horror stories of parents whose miscarried babies were whisked off to who-knows-where. Where do all these babies go? No one could answer my question. The term "medical waste" made my blood boil, and I found myself deeply angered by the injustice of it all: mothers made to leave the hospital with no closure whatsoever, no resting place to visit, no idea of where their child's remains ended up. It was — *is* — gruesome and wrong. I am deeply grateful for those on staff at our local hospital who tend to the special needs of grieving parents like my husband and me.

Fast-forward two years: I discovered that I was pregnant for the eighth time. For the first time in all my pregnancies, I found myself unable to relish the joy of an impending arrival. My heart was burdened by worry and anxiety. Miscarriage has a cruel way of robbing subsequent pregnancies of their joyful anticipation. Even though I had given birth to five healthy children, the fear of another loss loomed in my mind. Suddenly, I was aware of how scarred our losses had left me. But I fought to clear the dark clouds away and remain focused and positive, believing that we trend toward our most dominant thoughts.

I wish I could say that our eighth child is now with us. Sadly, exactly two years to the day after our traumatic loss of Xavier Paul, we found ourselves reliving the nightmare — only this time, I was already eighteen weeks pregnant.

Almost as devastating as seeing his still heart on the ultrasound screen was having to tell our five children that, once again, their tiny sibling had gone to Heaven. It tore my heart out. All of our children adore babies, and would gladly open their hearts to a dozen siblings. To say they were crushed is an understatement. Our thirteen-year-old son cried, while his eleven-year-old brother raged. Our daughter fled to her room and sobbed for an hour. She had wanted a sister so badly. Our two other sons sat in numb bewilderment. Grief has so many faces, and the pain of siblings who experience the untimely death of a brother or sister is real and often underestimated.

This time, I had a lovely new doctor who cared for me with a gentle compassion for which I will be forever grateful. She grieved along with me, and recognized the full and unique dignity of our baby. She couldn't tell me why he had died, but she walked me through the following days with the utmost sensitivity and grace. When those in the medical profession are open to being the hands and feet and voice of Christ, their work has the potential to heal on an even higher level than mere medicine.

After a long night of induced labor in the hospital, our eighth child, Blaise Mark, came into this world, his tiny eyes forever closed. After baptizing him, we were given the gift of precious time to hold him and say goodbye. The nurses wrapped him in a tiny blanket and miniature hat. Our children were allowed to visit and hold him, which was both beautiful and difficult. The nurses cried as our five-year-old son sadly asked if we couldn't just "give the baby some air."

Our previous experiences were more abstract in some ways; this one was real and raw. In many ways, it is uncharted territory. When an adult dies, there are expected and familiar traditions — a wake, a funeral, a burial. But a late-stage miscarriage feels like an odd gray area, with no set of rules or traditions.

In our case, we were able to have a funeral Mass for Blaise. We were once again blessed with the infant loss program offered by the hospital and were able to give him a proper burial. Blaise Mark was buried together with his brother Xavier, and they share a beautiful grave marker bearing both of their names. Being able to visit them and honor their memory is a treasure to our family — one that we wish was available for all parents who have walked this difficult path. It saddens us to see the names of families we know on nearby grave markers, whose children are also buried in this special area, but we know they, too, cherish the knowledge that their children's remains have a resting place until we can be reunited in eternal life.

Once again, the hard work of physical and emotional recovery began as life kept moving forward. As in the past, our faith carried us. People stepped forward to share their own stories of loss. The cards, meals, and compassionate words were touching and healing. Common suffering can bring people together for good, which is what we witnessed. While we were never able to adequately thank all the people who showed us such love, we took comfort in the knowledge that God sees all things and is never outdone in generosity.

A special word of recognition to a group that often goes unnoticed in the aftermath of miscarriage and infant loss: fathers. They hurt, too, although society often forgets this. My own husband, the father of our eight children, was a rock and source of steady strength throughout each of our losses — even while navigating his own grief. He cherished each of our tiny children as much as I did, and was deeply saddened by each loss.

While I cannot speak for the specific pain that a father feels at the death of his unborn child, there seems to be a double suffering for fathers: that of having to helplessly watch a beloved spouse endure such a difficult physical and emotional process. I cannot imagine what my husband went through when we lost our baby at ten weeks and I nearly bled to death on our bathroom floor. The instinct to protect is strong, and not being able to do so in such a situation is a heavy burden to bear. And unlike mothers, who often have fellow moms with whom to share their story and their pain, fathers more often are expected to move on and get back to the business of life. But they deserve our utmost compassion and understanding.

Finding healing after miscarriage looks different for each person. After our third loss, I was struck by the Scripture passage Job 1:21, which reminds us that the Lord giveth and the Lord taketh away. I felt keenly acquainted with this harsh reality, and yet somehow comforted by it. The most healing thought throughout all of our experiences was that we would someday be reunited with the children we never had the chance to know. And we will be granted an understanding of why we and so many others are asked to carry this heavy cross. Until that blessed day, we have faith that goodbye is not forever. That what the Lord has taken away will be restored.

CHAPTER 12

STILLBIRTH

Do You Trust My Son?

Sarah-Jean Ballard

I WAS RAISED IN a very anti-Catholic, Protestant home. Learning about Mary was the trickiest part of my conversion to the Catholic Faith. The more I learned about her, the more I realized how wrong all of my perceptions and beliefs were. Yet, even after seven years of being Catholic, it was still a point of discomfort for me, perhaps out of habit.

I never anticipated that she would make waves to change my relationship with her forever.

On May 2, 2022, Mary came to me in a vision while I was walking from one room to another in my house. Needless to say, I was in disbelief and quite troubled.

Mary suddenly appeared before me, standing on the ocean and yet right in front of me. It was as if the whole room went dark, and I could see that it was stormy off in the distance behind her. She spoke warmly but firmly and said to me, "Do you trust my Son?" to which I answered out loud, "Of course!" Then she said, "Do you trust me?" I hesitated, not wanting to answer her, but then humbled myself and quietly replied, "Of course ..." She looked serious and softly said, "A storm is coming and you need to trust Him and His plan for your life." And then, just as quickly as she had appeared, she was gone and the room was no longer dark.

I stood in disbelief for what felt like a long time, wondering if I had lost my mind. "*Maybe I'm working too hard? Maybe I should eat something? Maybe I didn't get enough sleep?!*" I thought to myself.

The next day, someone I follow on Instagram posted a picture of Mary, Star of the Sea (Stella Maris), and I had to catch my breath as I felt the goosebumps: I realized it was the same vision of Mary that I had, without ever having seen that picture before.

To me, that was confirmation that I wasn't insane and it really did happen. Still, I was afraid to even acknowledge the vision, since I didn't want anyone to think I was losing my mind. I didn't even tell my husband until much later. I was scared of the forewarning of her statement, even though I was supposed to "trust Him."

My immediate inclination was that I was going to suffer a miscarriage, even though I had never had that fear ever before in my life. Plus, I wasn't even pregnant! Or so I thought.

On May 5, 2022, I took a pregnancy test even though my period wasn't due for four more days and we were still trying to avoid pregnancy. I was not prepared for that second line to appear, but the immeasurable joy I felt upon seeing it was unlike any other time in my life. For the first time, I was filled with excitement and joyful anticipation rather than fear and anxiety as with my previous five pregnancies.

I waited until the next day to surprise my husband with the news, still in disbelief myself. To my surprise, he was just as excited and full of joy as I was! All of our other surprise pregnancies had always caused us so much anxiety, but this time felt different.

It made me forget all about my vision of Mary, at least for a couple of weeks.

Then the vision hit me around eight weeks into my pregnancy, and I immediately began to live in a constant state of fear, despite my promise to Mary that I would trust her Son. I started praying over my baby almost every night, hoping that everything would somehow turn out okay and that I wasn't insane for worrying about nothing.

When my mother-in-law became extremely ill and ultimately passed away, I hoped that was the storm I had been warned of. I waited for peace, but none came. I knew that wasn't my storm.

A once-solid friendship was also shattered, leaving behind the echoes of profound betrayal and the weight of a long-shared history that was now stained with pain and bitterness. I hoped that was the storm I was warned about, but the hardships continued.

My own mother's health started declining rapidly, and we received one bad report after another about her condition until she was in hospice with no hope of returning to a normal life. I desperately hoped that was the storm Mary warned me about, but I waited for God's reassurance and realized, once again, it wasn't over.

August 29, 2022 — Day 1

When I woke up on August 29, 2022, I had no idea it was going to be the worst day of my life.

I had no idea that when I put on my favorite white ruffled skirt, I would never be able to look at it the same way ever again.

I had no idea the next time I looked in my floor-length mirror, I would be coming to terms with the fact that my pregnant belly was the tomb of my dead baby.

I was *so* happy that I was going to finally see pictures of my baby at our twenty-week anatomy scan ultrasound! I was filled with joy thinking I would finally feel safe and know he was "okay" and could get ready to tell people about our newest addition that was on the way.

I felt like I had waited the whole four and a half months for this day to come, not knowing it would be the end.

The ultrasound tech started the scan, took a couple of pictures, and then said she had to go ask the doctor if those were the angles he wanted and quickly left the room. I immediately knew something was wrong. I looked at my husband and he looked back at me. "That's not good," he said. I nodded and said quietly, "I know."

She came back, pulled up my baby's chest on her screen, and took another picture. She then turned on the sound. And there was nothing. Where his heartbeat should be on the monitor, there was nothing. Time became a blur as she quickly hurried out of the room again without a word. I looked worried at my husband, and he looked more worried than I was. My heart started racing when I found no comfort in his face. I closed my eyes to stop the tears and started praying.

Suddenly the nurse came back with the doctor and they asked my husband and our other five children to go to the waiting room. A feeling of dread and panic washed over me. The doctor and ultrasound tech came back over to scan my belly again, both in silence. No one said anything. The silence was so awkward. I finally turned to the doctor and said, "So … what's happening?" He swallowed hard, tried to steady his voice, and said, "We can't find a heartbeat."

I felt like I stopped breathing. I stopped living in that moment, as if my own heartbeat wasn't there. This couldn't be real. It couldn't be happening. It must be a mistake.

But it wasn't. They continued to try to find his heartbeat, but there was only silence. They said they were going to call my health care provider so I could discuss what to do next, and then they walked out and left me alone. And I felt more alone than I've ever felt before. Like I was dead and the ultrasound room became my tomb.

When they finally came back, they told me they had contacted my midwife and that I could go see her immediately to discuss what to do next. I slowly got up, in a blur, void of all emotions. I didn't know what to think. I hadn't had time to process it.

As I walked down the hallway, all alone, my heart was racing and my thoughts were blank. The hallway couldn't have been more than fifteen feet to the exit, but it felt like it took forever to get to the door, as if it was the longest hallway in the world. When I finally reached the waiting room to meet my husband's worried gaze, I quickly said, "Okay, let's go," and started frantically searching for the elevator. He directed me and our five children toward the elevator. Once the doors shut, I blurted out, "They couldn't find a heartbeat." I don't remember what he said after that or what I said. Or if the kids said anything. Once those words came out of my mouth and my brain acknowledged what was going on, it all became a blur.

Then next thing I remember, we were all in the car, driving to my midwife's office. She told me all of my options and what would occur next. I felt extremely overwhelmed and unable to process anything she said. I appeared calm, but panic was overtaking every fiber of my being. I insisted she use the Doppler and try to find my baby's heartbeat, but it still wasn't there.

Once we got home, I tried to remain calm, but I was still in shock. And I was too scared to let myself come to terms with what was happening. It was all a blur.

August 30, 2022 — Day 2

I woke up at 5 a.m. in a cold sweat from a horrible nightmare. I sat straight up in bed with tears running down my face and realized all at once that it wasn't a dream. Rather, the nightmare I had was actually my reality. I started feeling short of breath, dizzy, while a surge of emotions washed over me. I quickly got out of bed and made my way downstairs into the kitchen, where I collapsed on the floor with an anxiety attack. I could barely breathe — I was choking on tears, shuddering, spitting, and shivering.

I cried for what felt like minutes, but I later realized it had been an hour and a half. I finally regained my breath and pulled myself together in time for my children to wake up.

I don't know how I made it through the day. I remember crying every so often and walking around in a daze, completely dead to the world.

I went into my walk-in closet to get a shirt, glanced over at the mirror, and noted that I still looked very much pregnant. This caused me to abruptly come to the realization that my dead baby was in my body. The last time I had looked in that mirror, I was smiling and rubbing my belly, admiring my outfit. Remembering that moment was a huge trigger for me and I collapsed again, sobbing more uncontrollably than I ever had before. My husband found me, held me, and sobbed with me.

Every time my husband found me sobbing, he cried with me. Somehow that made me feel even worse, because I felt so bad that I was the cause of him experiencing the same pain that I was experiencing. I felt like it was my fault, and I felt so bad for putting him through such immense pain, sadness, and loss. I never, *ever* wanted him to experience pain like this, and I couldn't help but feel that I was the cause.

I'm the baby maker. I'm the one who's supposed to make the babies. I felt like it was the only thing in my life I had ever done *right*. I felt like it was the only thing I was actually *good at*. So to have my faith and self-confidence blown right out the window was alarming, disheartening, and jarring.

Him crying with me, feeling the same pain, mourning the same loss — the loss of *our* son — it made it harder, and yet somehow easier. I didn't want him to experience that much pain, but knowing he knew and felt the same thing that I did was my only comfort. I've never felt so close to him, so connected to him, so unbelievably understood and validated. It was like we were finally of one mind and one body, in a way we had never been before.

August 31, 2022 — Day 3

We had to arrive at the hospital at 7:30 a.m. Fortunately, my niece was able to watch our five children all day.

My midwife met us at the hospital. There was no waiting. As soon as they saw me, they whisked us into the first empty room to start the process of inducing me.

I felt comforted knowing my midwife was there to support me through the entire process, just like she was for my other five deliveries. Supporting me, comforting me, hugging me, assuring me I would be okay.

My midwife knitted and talked, keeping me distracted for hours while we waited for the contractions to begin. Somewhere between 2 p.m. and 3 p.m. I started getting uncomfortable and shifting back and forth from the pain.

The following two hours became a blur, as usually happens in labor. It felt like five hours and also five minutes at the same time. I kept walking around as I normally would to encourage contractions, and also when it started getting rough. Then it hit me that I was in *labor* and was going to give birth to my dead baby, and I began to panic. My ears started ringing, my vision blurred, the room started to go black, and I knew I was going to pass out. I quickly lay down on the bed, on my left side, with my arm sticking out hanging off the side of the bed because of the IV in it, which had become increasingly sore and uncomfortable. I didn't move from that position again. I lay there, laboring with the contractions one on top of another, with little time to breathe between each one, and in my mind my thoughts were swirling.

I realized I was going to give birth to my baby, and I couldn't stop it. For the first time in my life, I didn't *want* to give birth. I didn't want the baby to come out. I didn't want it to be over. One contraction after another, like a wave, rushing over me. And then I finally felt the widespread surge through my body, as I have many times before, and

I knew it was time. I pulled my dress out of the way and shifted slightly, which apparently was enough for others in the room to realize it was time and come to catch the baby.

In that moment, I tried to fight what was happening because I suddenly realized it was almost over. And I would rather suffer through more contractions than let my baby leave my body. It was as if my brain knew he wasn't supposed to come out yet.

One more big contraction rushed over me and I realized he was coming out whether I pushed or not. So I did nothing. I was still lying on my side, face buried in the bed. For the first time while laboring, I lay there and did absolutely nothing, knowing my body would do what it had to do. And it did. It happened without me having to move. Without having to push. He came out all at once, "en caul" (with the amniotic sac intact), placenta attached, all in one piece.

Dylan Marinus was born at 6:43 p.m.

As soon as he left my body, I started to sob loudly and violently, only stopping briefly to ask if everything came out okay and if I was all right and if he was "okay."

The two nurses and my midwife assured me that he was "fine," and I realized later that was such a stupid question.

I wept uncontrollably for over forty-five minutes while my husband and my midwife hugged me, held me, cried with me, and comforted me. In the back of my mind, I wanted to see Dylan, but I knew he was still safe in the amniotic sac. So I kept crying.

Once I was finally able to stop crying, I sat up and asked for my baby. I didn't know what to expect. I had never seen a dead baby before. Nothing really prepares you for that moment. But there he was. My tiny baby. Perfectly formed fingers, a nose like his other brothers, soft hair, and his daddy's feet.

They called a priest to come and bless Dylan immediately after birth and pray with us. I cried the entire time, holding Dylan, who was carefully swaddled in a tiny blanket with sea turtles on it that the hospital had provided.

Hours passed and they urged me to go home, but I didn't want to leave him. I wasn't ready to say goodbye. Four hours with Dylan wasn't long enough.

I was so conflicted. I was grateful they said I could go home and I didn't have to sleep there, but I also didn't want to leave him! I didn't want to leave my baby, knowing I would never see him again until I get to Heaven. Hugging him, saying goodbye to him, and having to walk away without him was absolutely the worst, most horrible, most painful thing I've ever had to do in my life.

September 1, 2022 — Day 4

We continued crying and mourning the loss of Dylan all day. I don't even remember sleeping that night. I might have cried all night long.

With so little sleep and so much trauma, it felt like a Herculean task waiting to hear for autopsy results, blood work results, dealing with the funeral home, finding out what our burial options were, deciding who to call and notify about what had happened. All of this while taking care of our children, who were also navigating the grief and horror of what we had gone through.

September 2, 2022 — Day 5

My heart felt like it was just going to stop beating from the pain — like I could just die from hurting so much. My husband felt it too.

But unlike him, I was also *angry*.

Angry that I wouldn't wear maternity clothes anymore.

Angry when I saw on my laundry pile the nursing clothes that I wouldn't get to wear now.

Angry that I wouldn't be able to use the newborn clothes I had just bought and washed for him.

Angry that I was overweight and wouldn't even get a baby to kiss and love and hold in exchange.

Angry that I couldn't do anything to stop him from dying.

Angry that I had no control. I couldn't stop it from happening. I couldn't keep him. I couldn't keep him in my body. *Angry that I was forced to let go of something I didn't want to let go of.*

Angry that no one on this earth would ever love Dylan more than my husband and I did.

September 5, 2022 — Day 8

I can't put into words that whole first week after losing my baby. I spent most days crying with my husband, barely surviving. Our children caught a cold, and it made everything so much harder. I remember asking earlier that day how it could possibly get any worse. And then it did.

My brother called me at 11:00 p.m. to tell me that our mom had passed away.

On some level, I was prepared to lose my mother, so when it actually happened, it felt surreal, and I wasn't even sure how to process it. That moment will forever be etched in my heart though, not just for the profound loss of my mother, but for another reason. As soon as I hung up the phone, my husband immediately grabbed our children, gathered them around, put his arms around me, and proceeded to lead us in prayer, asking for the repose of her soul and God's mercy upon her at the moment of her death. That moment touched me in ways I'll never be able to explain fully. That was a deeply moving and profound testament to my husband's heart.

I had been so caught up in my own emotions, still trying to process the loss of my son, that admittedly it might have taken awhile before I even thought of that. Yet, in the midst of him experiencing the same loss as me, he still knew that praying for her soul was the most important thing to do in that moment. That really made a profound impact on me.

In the days and weeks following the loss of my son, and then my mother, I struggled through many dark and empty days. I cried myself to sleep every night and woke up every morning hoping it was all a bad dream, but quickly realizing that it wasn't. Getting through each day felt like an unbearable burden.

I struggled greatly between begging God to console me and giving in to overwhelming feelings of bitterness. I kept asking Him *why* He let this happen to *me*.

Some days I was able to pray and other days I wasn't. Many days I struggled with so much anger and bitterness that I couldn't talk to God at all. And other times, I was able to pray a Rosary, but couldn't form thoughts or words of my own to plead with God from my heart.

The roller coaster of grief was unlike anything I had ever experienced before, and so much of it, I realize now, I have blocked out of my memory. I felt completely unprepared to deal with such intense loss and trauma. It feels completely impossible to process all the thoughts and emotions from losing a child. No one should ever have to say goodbye to their child. How can anyone really be prepared to process such a thing?

Yet Mary did.

Everyone responds to pain, loss, and trauma differently—there's no one single way to deal with grief. The hardest part for me was accepting that I had no control over what happened, nor did I have any control over my grief journey or the amount of time it would take to recover. I struggled greatly with impatience over how long it was taking me to heal from the pain.

Four months after losing my son, I became extremely frustrated and angry that I was still so broken, so sad, so empty, and so *lifeless*. I grieved not only the loss of my son but the loss of my life's story taking a turn that I never intended. I was filled with so much anger and resentment over the fact that I was now "the girl whose baby died" and I couldn't fix my story.

My situation was made worse by feeling abandoned by family and friends. No one tells you that you'll be grieving not only for your child but for the loss of friendships of people who don't know how to support you through that sadness. I think too many people don't want to acknowledge miscarriage, stillbirth, or infant loss because they can't fathom going through it themselves and so they have no idea how to support someone who finds themselves in that horrible club that no one wants to be in.

The only consolation I found was in my newfound friends who had also experienced miscarriage, stillbirth, or infant loss. It was equally heartbreaking to find other people suffering as much as I was, and yet comforting to know I wasn't alone.

When Lent began, I remember the entire notion of Lenten sacrifices felt like a cruel joke. I remember seeing posts on social media about the things that people would "give up for Lent," like chocolate, extra snacks, or coffee. I scoffed at all of it, thinking how meaningless and trivial these small sacrifices really were in the grand scheme of things. I had to give up my baby! There could be no bigger sacrifice than that, right?

Someone finally said something to me that brought me comfort in the midst of those thoughts about Lenten sacrifice. She said, "Sometimes we choose our Lent, and sometimes God chooses our Lent for us."

And that made me realize that I didn't need to dream up a sacrifice for Lent. One had already been chosen for me, and my job was to unite my suffering with His. I continued to learn how to do that every day going forward. As we struggled to conceive again, the call to relinquish my need for control became even more apparent. Nothing is more humbling than being continually reminded that ultimately you are not in control of the things you once thought you were. It was a hard lesson, which I was growing more resistant to and more resentful of each day.

When we finally got a positive pregnancy test in April, I felt relieved and had a great sense of triumph, as if I had finally accomplished something! I had worked so hard at tracking my cycles and timing everything perfectly. I felt so proud that I had achieved my goal. When the lines on the pregnancy tests didn't get any darker after three days, I began panicking and went for blood work to have my HCG levels checked. Hours before we got the results of that blood test I started bleeding, and we lost our seventh baby after only five days of being aware of his or her existence. We will never know for sure whether that baby was a boy or a girl, but I decided to name *her* anyway. Shay Angelica, pray for us.

And that is when I finally hit rock bottom. Losing Dylan was horrible. Having trouble conceiving again was horrible. The sad ending to my attempt at conceiving my rainbow baby was horrible. *All of it was just horrible.* I felt like I had nothing left to live for. It was definitely one of the darkest times for me in my grief journey.

And that's when I finally learned to *let go*.

Mary said to Gabriel, "Behold, I am the handmaid of the Lord; let it be to me according to your word" (Luke 1:38).

Once again, I found that the profound example of Mary's ability to just *let go and let God* somehow helped scrape what was left of me off the floor, lift me up, and help me go on.

After losing Dylan, I realized that I had become angry and resentful of Mary. She had warned me about the suffering that I would endure, and I know they say, "Don't shoot the messenger," but her alerting me of the sorrows that were to come felt mean rather than helpful. Something suddenly made me realize that I had to stop being angry at her and let her back into my life. So that's what I did for the whole month of May, the month honoring Mary. And I don't think that was a coincidence.

By the end of May, I found myself finally willing to submit to God's will for my life, whatever that might be. I realized that worrying every single second that I wasn't going to be able to conceive any more children wasn't going to change anything. Worrying never actually helps anyone. Living in fear doesn't do us any favors. That's why God commands us 365 times between Genesis and Revelation to not be afraid. Why then do we feel such a strong need to live in the state of fear instead of trusting God?

Mary is the ultimate example of fully surrendering to God's will, completely submitting to His plans, and living without fear. At so many different points, Mary had every reason to be afraid. But she chose not to. She chose the hard path of complete and total surrender to God's will, even when it was scary and didn't make sense. Mary's fearlessness stuck out to me in a way that it never had before. She made me realize that's what I had to do, no matter how hard it seemed.

On May 31, the feast of the Visitation made a profound impression on me, leaving me with a sense of peace that I didn't have before. Realizing how God had worked miracles in both Mary's and Elizabeth's lives and wombs gave me hope. It was the first time I had truly felt *hope* in my future, and a painting of the Visitation, with unsurpassed joy on Mary's and Elizabeth's faces, has brought me so much comfort from that day forward.

I think the hardest part of everyone's grief journey is setting aside fear and learning how to have hope again. That will look different for each individual person, but for me, Mary was my beacon of inspiration on my journey.

Mary proved once again to play an integral and important part in my healing. On August 15, the feast of the Assumption of Mary into Heaven, she prompted me to take a pregnancy test just minutes before walking out the door for Mass that day. Imagine my surprise when a faint second line appeared! I laughed out loud because it felt providential. I quickly ran downstairs to find my husband and make him look at the test to assure me that I wasn't imagining things. He confirmed what I saw, and we were both filled with cautious hope for the future and a sense of peace that we didn't have last time. Something felt profoundly different this time.

It took nearly one year from losing Dylan to be able to find that glimmer of hope in the midst of our grief.

I suddenly realized that many milestones along that road somehow seemed to align with the Church year.

First, pondering the significance of the Immaculate Conception and Mary's "Let it be to me according to your word" in response to the angel Gabriel taught me the response all of us need to have when it comes to God's plan for our life. Her yes to being the Mother of God literally changed history forever.

Then, during Lent especially, I reflected on how Mary had to say yes again by giving that Baby back to the Father in the worst imaginable way possible — watching Jesus die on the Cross. How our loss pales in comparison to hers, doesn't it?

After that, reflecting on the feast of the Visitation helped me realize that God makes all things possible, as He did for Elizabeth. Even John the Baptist, within his mother's womb, could experience joy and hope for the future.

And so it felt not only poetic but providential to learn on the feast day of the completion of Mary's mission on earth, the Assumption, that God was going to bless us with another child.

It was only after pondering those milestones that I was finally able to connect all the dots and realize how important Mary had been on my entire journey. She was there all along. And of course she was! She is the one in the Nursery of Heaven after all. She's the one who's holding, cuddling, and caring for all our babies that left us too soon. She knows the pain of losing a child better than anyone else, so she can intimately comfort us through our own experiences of loss more so than any other person after her Son.

Our babies are not lost forever. They are in the Nursery of Heaven, waiting for us, praying for us, and longing to comfort us until we can one day be reunited.

Dylan Marinus and Shay Angelica, pray for us.

CHAPTER 13

Stillbirth

Silent Night

Sarah Tafoya

It was December 27, 2016. My husband and I had just dropped off the kids at my in-laws with a promise to come back with tacos in a couple of hours, after an appointment with my ob-gyn. My due date was December 22, but both of my other children were born a week and a half late, so I just assumed the same would be the case for this child. We had found out the gender of both my daughter and son, so we had decided to be surprised with this baby.

I remember shifting uncomfortably in the car as one does when she is nine months pregnant and ready to hang the eviction notice up. My husband and I talked about what day we thought the doctor would suggest inducing if this became necessary. He grabbed a coffee and we went into the waiting room. I did the whole shebang—peed in a cup, got my blood pressure and weight taken, and so on. Then the doctor came in to check the heartbeat.

He had difficulty finding it. He kept moving the instrument around, assuming that the baby was in a weird position, trying not to alarm me or my husband. Finally he said, "We will need to do an ultrasound."

Pause here for a second. Previously, every time the doctor had done this, he found my baby's heartbeat almost instantly without any searching, so I knew something was wrong. I am an optimist by nature, though, so I figured that maybe the machine was not working right. I was trying to grasp any explanation other than what I knew was the rational one.

The doctor then performed the ultrasound, but he again could not find the heartbeat. He hesitated. He knew our child had passed, but he did not want to tell us — and we knew our child had passed, but we did not want to hear him say it either. He then checked everything — fluids, organs, placenta. Everything was perfect. Nothing was out of the ordinary.

He asked, "When did you last feel movement?" My husband remembered that, on Christmas night, the baby had been going bonkers moving around. That was the last time I had felt a lot of movement. The day after Christmas, we had gone out to dinner to celebrate our niece's birthday, and I remember feeling an uncomfortable shift of body weight from the upper part of my belly to the lower part. Had there been other times? My memory is not that great, and I am not a worrier by nature. So I wasn't really keeping track of how often I was feeling movement. There is not a lot of room for them to be squirming around anyway.

The doctor said he would induce that day, so we would be able to know more about what had happened. He explained, "Often, the most active kids can get themselves into trouble and twist up the umbilical cord." This kid was definitely active, so I would not be surprised. The doctor called the hospital and said he would meet us there.

Leaving the doctor's office that day was one of the most awkward things I have ever done. Everyone knew what had happened. But they were so caring, and they promised to pray for us and our family. It was so strange, though. Thirty minutes before, I was excited to give birth and eat tacos but now everything had been turned on its head. I didn't have any words. Neither did my husband. "I guess we'll have to tell your mom we're not getting tacos," I managed to blurt out.

I called my mom to let her know we were heading to the hospital, but not for the reason we were expecting. I am sure it was one of the worst calls she had ever received. She certainly wasn't expecting to hear, "Mom, they couldn't find a heartbeat. We are being induced." I don't even remember saying those words, but I know they came out of my mouth. Shock is the only thing that gets you through those moments, because otherwise I probably wouldn't have been able to breathe, let alone speak. Our parents spread the word to our siblings, who made plans to meet us at the hospital.

When we arrived, we made our way up to the labor and delivery floor. Our nurses were awesome. Not one to deal with tragedy well, I kept up a good banter with them as they admitted me and hooked me up to receive Pitocin. When this formality was over, my husband and I were left alone in the room for the first time. I remember holding his hand. Squeezing it, not sure what or how he was feeling. We still didn't know if our baby was a boy or a girl. While my husband always thinks we are having a boy, somewhere deep inside I was sure it was a girl. We both cried. It finally hit us that our precious baby was not going to be coming home with us. This was really happening.

A hospital representative came to us and asked about funeral plans and other things you have to think about when you are the parent of a child who has passed. The reality of what was happening was starting to sink in. This was happening, whether we wanted to deal with it or not. After she left they began the induction using Pitocin. They weren't sure how long it would take. It all depended on how my body would react. My mother and youngest sister arrived shortly after. We all sobbed, hugged one another, and talked over what we knew so far. After about an hour, my husband's mom and sister arrived as well. My dad came next, followed by my other sister, who was six months pregnant, and her husband. My mom called our parish priest, who said he would come as soon as he could.

Things were progressing well, so they broke my water. At this point, I decided to get the epidural. Everyone left, and they administered it. The doctor told me that I was at ten centimeters and that when I felt a push to go with it. My husband grabbed one of my legs, and the nurse held the other. After two big pushes, I felt a giant relief, the child leaving my body. That is always such a wonderful feeling; the feeling that something amazing just happened. The fruition of nine months of waiting has finally come to an end.

Then I felt a rush of emotions. A lot of things had been swirling around in my head during the labor process. Was it a boy or a girl? What would he or she look like? Would he or she have hair? (All my babies were born with a full head of hair.) How long had the child been in my womb after the umbilical cord had been twisted? Was that what had caused him or her to pass? I was about to have answers. In reality, everything happens in a matter of seconds, but it seems to be in slow motion. "You have a beautiful daughter," the doctor said. He wrapped her and handed her to me and my husband. She looked perfect. Beautiful, dark black hair, delicate features, ten fingers and ten toes. Dark red lined her lips and tinted her fingernails. Everything you would expect from a newborn. The doctor examined the umbilical cord, and sure enough there was a large kink in it. He estimated that she might have passed within the previous twelve to twenty-four hours. Everything else seemed to be normal. That was the only logical explanation. They weighed her and got her measurements and cleaned up the room and then the anxious family outside was allowed to enter.

It was strange, because even though her spirit was no longer with her body, I was still excited to show her off to everyone. Through the tears, I could sense that others felt the same way. Even though it was for the briefest of moments, she was . . . no, she *is* an important member of our family. She continues to be. Everyone held her and had their picture taken with her. Then our family priest arrived and baptized her. We named her Isabel Lucia. Isabel is a derivative of Elizabeth, my mother's name and my middle name, and Lucia (Lucy) was my husband's paternal grandmother's name and my sister's middle name. The priest encouraged us and those present to make the Sign of the Cross on her forehead and hold her. We sang "Silent Night." Since that moment, it has become her song, at least in my mind. The words "sleep in heavenly peace" are now difficult to choke out as they directly link me to that moment in the hospital when the whole family gently sang to my daughter and I stroked her cheek. An hour or so later, everyone began to head home. By then, it was 9 p.m., and everyone was emotionally drained. It was a hard drive home for our parents and siblings. It was soon to be the toughest night of my life.

The nurse took Isabel into the other room. They were going to give her a bath and clean her up so she looked her best while we got some rest. My husband settled in to the fold-out bed and turned on the TV. While there was nothing good on, I don't think he could have handled the silence. Eventually, he fell asleep. But I could not. Too much was still swirling around in my head. The floodgates officially opened, and I cried the entire night. I had been able to keep it together for most of the day, but everything finally caught up with me. In my solitude, I was able to really let myself feel what had happened during the course of the day. I had just lost a child. This was really happening.

I had been blindsided. No one saw it coming. I had never heard of someone going full-term and then losing a child when there were no complications along the way. This was all new territory. I had lost people in my life, but no one ever this close. I guess it is hard to imagine until you experience it. A child is literally part of you, so losing him or her hits you in a different way from anyone else.

I cried to sort out my feelings. I cried as I thought about my family and the sorrow they were feeling. I cried because my husband and I would have to find some way to explain to our other two children that they would not have a little sister to play with. The list in my head of things that would not be the way I had imagined kept growing. Then a friend texted me to ask how the pregnancy was going and if I would be going into labor soon. I just stared at the screen for a while, not sure how I wanted to respond. Should I tell her what had happened? Could I even type the words? "Just had a baby girl, she twisted her umbilical cord and was stillborn." I waited. Should I rephrase it? There is really no good way to tell someone bad news like this. I sent it. Words of comfort were sent my way. I managed to text someone from my work and let them know what had happened. They would need to know, after all. Again it was hard to write the words. There was a knot in my throat.

Tears continued to roll down my cheeks throughout the night, as I found it difficult to sleep or think of anything else. Then a thought entered my mind. I should pray. I started the Chaplet of Divine Mercy. I stumbled upon it after college when I was hired to do production for a Catholic radio station. I loved the simplicity of the Chaplet and the comfort it gives with its emphasis on God's unfathomable mercy. It was really its closing prayer, though, that hooked me: "Eternal God, in whom mercy is endless and the treasury of compassion inexhaustible, look kindly upon us and increase your mercy in us, that in difficult moments we might not despair, nor become despondent, but with great confidence submit ourselves to your holy will, which is Love and Mercy itself." Jesus, I trust in you.

In difficult moments, we pray that we might not despair but submit to God's holy will. This was that difficult moment, the most difficult one in my life up to that point. This was the prayer I needed most that night. I kept repeating, "Lord, help me to submit to Your will, help me to accept Your will." I do not believe that God took Isabel away from us or that He caused her to twist her umbilical cord, but I do believe that He will use her death for something powerful. He already has, as I am here sharing her story. No, I was not angry at God that night, nor am I angry at Him today. Thankfully, I was saved from such thoughts. I know that every life has a purpose. I know that my daughter is a powerful intercessor for our family, and I know that God uses every single thing in our lives, good or bad, for a greater purpose. Slowly, as time goes on, I am seeing some of His plan.

Back to that night, though. After I prayed for a while, a nurse came to check on me. When I asked her the time, she said it was 3:40 a.m. That is when I received my first sign that everything was going to be okay. I had no idea when I had begun praying, but I then found out that I had started at the hour of Divine Mercy — three o'clock. Boom. A sign from God that He was there with me, nudging me closer to Him through the tears. This was my "Footprints in the Sand" moment. It was still tough the rest of the night, but I knew I was not alone. God had my back. So I continued to pray for trust, for patience, and for guidance.

The next morning, we asked that Isabel be brought to our room and we took turns holding and snuggling her. I just remember her being so cold, which is understandable, but the mother in me kept trying to warm her in some way. The nurse came to tell us that the photographer from the hospital was there and wanted to know if we wanted pictures. We said yes. Isabel got pictures taken by herself, and then we were allowed to be in the pictures. These would be our very last moments physically holding her. I could barely keep it together emotionally. I have the worst memory in the world, so the only thing going through my mind the entire time was, "Don't forget, never forget," as if by saying this multiple times I might magically be able to remember forever. I didn't want to let her go. Who would? This beautiful little child was mine. I didn't want God to take her, yet I knew that He already had — and that He was giving me a great opportunity to trust Him. So we released her, kissed her goodbye, and hugged one another tightly.

As we drove to my in-laws' house to pick up the kids, the car felt very empty. To our surprise, when we walked into their house, neither of our children even noticed my lack of belly. We took them home and broke the news. The hospital had given us a pamphlet and books, but none of them said exactly what we felt needed to be said, so we just winged it. There weren't any tears at first. I think it took awhile to sink in for them. Over the course of the next few days, my daughter asked more questions and cried in my lap. She was five, my son three. To them it was mostly a concept. Mom is "having" a baby. They couldn't see the baby or hear the baby, so it was just words, and then when I was not "having" a baby, again it was words. They never saw Isabel in person. She wasn't a physical reality to them, but that didn't mean she didn't leave a mark on their lives. There were moments of pain in their eyes and hearts, when they questioned why she had to die. Those are the hardest moments, as your grief combines with theirs.

Miraculously, I found a book at the library that talked about a baby in the womb and how its guardian angel is there to help them. At the end of the book, the angel remarks that soon the baby will go into the world and, when it is time, the angel would guide the child to a much bigger world. I love this because it gave comfort to me as well as to the children. To think that our guardian angel, even when we cannot see it, is always there to guide us from our birth to Heaven is an amazing thought.

Over the following days, my husband and I set out to do something we never imagined ourselves doing — planning a funeral for our child. We got everything settled at the funeral home, bought a burial plot for each of us (Isabel is in my gravesite and will be with me once I pass), and talked with our parish priest about a funeral Mass. Those days flew by as we surrounded ourselves with both sides of our family for meals and snuggled with the kids in our bed at night. We also planned a three-day getaway for the day after the funeral.

The funeral was a whirlwind. It was full of emotion, not just for us but for everyone present. I was surprised by how many came. I had broken the news on Facebook only earlier in the day. The only people who knew about Isabel's passing were those who had heard by word of mouth. For a child only a handful of people had met, there were so many people who mourned. I did well, only tearing up a couple of times during the Mass. My husband, my father, and I each spoke about Isabel during the funeral Mass. It was good to give her a loving send-off and to speak from the heart about what she meant to us. Afterward, we traveled to the cemetery. At the end of the priest's words, people began to head back to their cars. The moment that broke me was when my son yelled out, "I want my baby!" All I could do was hold him and say, "Me too!"

Dealing with the loss of a child is not something I ever expected to be experiencing in my thirties. While it took my husband and me by surprise, we have been able to move forward. There are moments when the loss will overtake you. Don't fight it. It is okay. It is healthy. My sister soon gave birth to her baby girl. As I went to the hospital to see the baby, I didn't know how I would feel. But I was able to hold her and snuggle her without any issues. On the drive home, however, I cried the whole way. I found myself re-mourning my daughter, the playmate my niece would have had.

These feelings remained with me for days, until my sister's milk came in and the baby was not latching. My sister needed my help. Once I was able to go and help her, I could refocus my pain and make it useful. There are times when I look at my niece (who is also my godchild) and think, "*Is this what Isabel would have been like?*" I know, of course, that each child is unique, and that Isabel would have her own personality and appearance. But they would have been very close in age. So when my niece is playing with my three children, there is a part of me that imagines how well Isabel would have enjoyed her siblings, and my niece sometimes plays that role in my head. I really try not to go there, because it can take you to the "what if" game — a game that never ends and can be as dark as a rabbit hole — but it does happen on occasion. I sometimes wonder if my older two treat my niece like the little sister they do not have. They watch out for her the way they would a younger sibling, and my son especially adores her. You would think, "*What do little kids know about loss?*" but they really seem to have a grip on it. Maybe more than I do at times. They understand the emptiness left by Isabel.

My husband and I talk about Isabel with the children. Often they talk about her on their own, my daughter especially. They pray to her. There are times when my children will break down and cry about how they miss their sister, even now, three years later. This can and will spark something in my own heart. I am not very good with emotion, so this is the part where I want to jump ship, but since they are so sensitive, listening to them and recognizing they are real people with real emotional concerns really helps me to face the emotions I am feeling. I talk and sometimes cry along with them. I tell them it is okay to miss their sister.

For me it has been helpful to have pictures of Isabel around the house. It is proof of her existence and establishes a physical place for her in our family. There is a picture of her at both my parents' and my in-laws' houses. Again, she is with us and a part of our family, even without her physical presence. I know not all families would be on board with this and some might think it strange. "Can't you just move on? Why are you constantly reminding yourself of loss?" That is one way to look at it, but I am never sad to see Isabel's picture. It comforts me to see her, as it would to see any picture of a loved one who has passed. We go to the cemetery to visit Isabel as a family and say a prayer. We go on her birthday and on some special occasions or whenever the kids ask. They asked a lot during the first year. My daughter likes to include Isabel in holiday celebrations. She always makes a Valentine for her and draws pictures for her.

In the days that followed Isabel's funeral, my husband and I discussed having another child. We were both eager to become pregnant again. God helped us to work on patience first. It took us six months. I know that is not terribly long, but when you are hoping every day to be with child, as I know many are, a month seems like forever. Every time a pregnancy test is taken and comes back negative or your period starts, there is a sense of failure, a thought that your prayers have fallen on deaf ears. This is what it feels like, but when you look at these events in hindsight, you see God's gentleness saying, "The answer is not no, but not yet. When the time is right, my child, you will see." God has the perfect family in store for you. Moments like this remind us that our plan is not God's plan, and while it seems trite, it is so true that sometimes only the experience of life and reflection can bring this truth to light in our minds.

It has been three years since Isabel's passing. In that time, many things have happened. My sister had a baby girl whose umbilical cord was around her neck but was born perfectly healthy. Her middle name is Isabel. We now have another beautiful son, born fifteen months after Isabel. His existence is proof of God's plan at work, as I know for a fact that my husband and I would not have worked so hard to have a child if we'd had a newborn in the house. He is a great blessing to our family, and I cannot imagine our life without him. Without taking the place of Isabel, he has helped us to move forward.

Since Isabel, I have heard from coworkers and family friends about their experience with miscarriage or stillbirth. It has made me aware that infant loss happens to many. We all belong to a big club that no one wanted access to, but together we find comfort in sharing the lives of our children. Our family has been struck with the passing of several relatives over the past couple of years. For me and my children, it has been easier to deal with the loss of our loved ones, knowing that they are now with Isabel.

I try to explain to my children that our life is like a giant puzzle. When you start, you only have a couple of pieces together and it looks like a big mess, but God knows what the entire, wonderful puzzle looks like. This is why we need to trust Him. This is difficult for me to do sometimes, but I am starting to see some of the pieces coming together in retrospect.

When I found out I was pregnant with Isabel, I went to a new doctor. The practice I had gone to before was perfectly fine, but something called me to this doctor, who was a faithful, practicing Catholic. After Isabel passed, I realized that God guided me to this doctor and his practice knowing what would happen and that I would need that kind of support.

I try to be open about Isabel with others who ask. I know that I am not required to share, and I know that not everyone is able to talk as freely as I am, but I also know that being open about my experience is something that can be strengthening for others who have been in a similar situation. God created us for community and we thrive when we embrace it.

My daughter will always be loved and remembered. She is proof that every life, even ones cut short, have purpose and meaning in this world.

If you are experiencing the loss of a child, I recommend five things:

Pray. Get all of your emotions out to God. If you are angry, fearful, or sad, let it out.

Trust. Hand everything over to God. This is easy to say but difficult to do. Keep at it.

Cling to your spouse and let him or her know what you are feeling. You may grieve differently. This is okay. Keeping your feelings to yourself does not work.

Let others help you. Whether it is time for talk, a meal, or just prayer, we are a community for a reason. God wants us to help others.

Do something for someone else. When we are charitable, it can help us get out of a funk.

CHAPTER 14

STILLBIRTH

Always a Part of Me

Dominic Tafoya

THE PREGNANCY WITH ISABEL was different for me than it was for my first daughter and my son. I had just finished graduate school and held a position at a hospital, which allowed me to take time off without having to worry about how much I would have to make up when I returned. I was truly excited to get away from the hospital to enjoy quality time with my new baby. Actually, I treated Isabel like my trophy. I had finished my master's degree in October and she was my reward to come in December. When she didn't come, I felt cheated, to say the least.

The day started off so great. It was one of my first days of paternity leave, as the baby was due anytime. I remember leaving that morning to go to Sarah's doctor's appointment to discuss how far along she was and possibly set up a time to induce her because she was overdue. On the way to her doctor's office, Sarah and I discussed what we were going to do for lunch and even stopped at Starbucks because we were early.

When we arrived at the office, Sarah went through all the routine things, such as answering the nurse's questions about how she was feeling and being weighed. Next on the docket was having an ultrasound to hear the baby's heartbeat. The nurse strapped the ultrasound pad to her belly and started the test, but could find no heartbeat. She thought that maybe the baby was positioned in a way that muffled her heartbeat, but after a few tries, she was still unsuccessful. The doctor then came and put us in a different room, where there was a 3-D ultrasound machine. Sarah was strapped to the machine, but once again no heartbeat could be heard. The doctor tried maneuvering the probe but to no avail, and he said, "I am really sorry, guys," several times. At first I didn't grasp that his apology was for us losing the baby. Then I came to the unnerving realization that our baby was gone. I went into shock. This could not be happening to us. Sarah got dressed, and the doctor told us that he would make arrangements at the hospital for Sarah to be induced. As we got into the car to head to the hospital, Sarah said we should call everyone to tell them what was going on. By this time I was numb and just going through the motions of what we had to do next. I could not fully grasp what was going on.

The first person I called was my mother. I told her the horrible news that our baby was gone and that I was taking Sarah to the hospital to be induced. I let her know I would tell her more once we got there. Before I hung up with her, I remember her saying, "I am so sorry, Dominic," and I said, "Me too." Sarah called her mom before we arrived at the hospital. Once we got settled in our room, Sarah and I were finally alone to discuss what was going on and what was going on in our minds. This was the first time I had ever cried so emotionally as an adult. I told Sarah I was not sure I could handle knowing if our baby was a boy or a girl; at that point, I didn't want to know and just wanted to leave.

After they induced Sarah and she gave birth to our beautiful daughter Isabel, the doctor noticed the umbilical cord was kinked and said that this was most likely the cause of her death. After Sarah gave birth, my mom and sister and Sarah's mom and dad and the rest of her family were there to visit. The priest who had married us and baptized our other children was kind enough to drive to the hospital that night and baptize Isabel.

When we were getting ready to leave the next day, I told Sarah I thought it would be nice for the kids and us to get away for a few days after Isabel's funeral. When we got home, we stopped at my parents' house to pick up the kids. My mom asked if I needed anything and what I wanted most was to be surrounded by family for a few days, which was the only thing I thought would bring me any sort of comfort, and it did. The next few days my family and I were either at my parents' house or at my in-laws' from around lunchtime to after dinner. I was afraid that if I was left alone too long my thoughts would take me over and I would become depressed, so being around family for the majority of the day really helped. I was able to be myself and express my emotions without being judged — and to hear how people in the family were affected by Isabel's death. The support from both sides of the family and from our friends was just so overwhelming. I am forever grateful.

After a few days, I needed to call my daughter's school, because we had been planning to move her from three days a week to five days after the baby came, so I had to notify them that she would be staying at three days. When I spoke to the receptionist, she said how sorry she was to hear of Isabel's passing and that she was surprised how uplifted I sounded. I remember telling her that either I could be a complete jerk or I could continue to be myself, and I knew the second was what Isabel would have wanted. I told her it helped that family had been there for us, helping us cope with our terrible loss.

It was so crazy to have to convince people that I was doing okay. People at work would come up to me months after Isabel had passed and let me know they were thinking or praying for me. So much support and kindness shown toward us made it easier to be at peace and to move forward.

Everyone handles grief differently. For me, having family with me when I needed them most, whether it was just to talk on the phone or to see each other, was a big help in getting me through it. From day one, Sarah and I agreed that anytime we wanted or needed to talk about Isabel, we would do so without reservation. That really helped then, and it does to this day. I know that if I have a dream, thought, or memory about Isabel, I can open up to her about it without feeling that I could potentially make her feel sad, and she knows that she can do the same with me. My advice to anyone going through something like this would be to have this "open-door" policy to speak. Since we do grieve differently, even in marriage, it is important to be open to your spouse about what you are feeling so that you can support one another and not drift apart.

There are times when I think, "*What if we had induced Sarah earlier? What would life actually be like having Isabel with us?*" I try not to go there because I know I cannot change the past. Wondering what would have been doesn't help anyone. I make it a point to think about her every day, but what I don't do is wonder what she would be like at any given age. She will always be a part of me and with me, and for that I am forever grateful to her.

CHAPTER 15

Stillbirth

Learning to Accept Uncertainty

Theoni Bell

As we sped through an intersection, I turned to my children with an anxious smile and told them, "It's going to be okay. We're just meeting the baby early. She will be in the NICU for a while, but she'll be so tiny and cute." At the hospital, I left my family in the car and went in to meet my baby alone. Covid regulations restricted anyone from coming with me. All I had was the green rosary wrapped around my wrist.

I was about seven months along in my pregnancy, and every single marker in every single ultrasound or lab was good. I had started experiencing achiness and fatigue four days earlier. It increased to intense, shooting pains in my hips, back, and groin. I thought I was just carrying too much weight and not moving around enough, so I took my kids on walks. On December 3, 2020, I finally called my doctor and realized I was having contractions! My husband, Bastian, took me to the hospital immediately.

After I had been pacing in the hallway behind a small window for ten minutes, a nurse in a face mask opened the double doors and I was finally allowed to enter the maternity wing. Still alone, but excited to meet my baby, I was strapped with a fetal monitor around my waist. The ultrasound technician began searching the screen, repositioning me, and frowning. She called a nurse to confirm what she was seeing, and they told me there was no heartbeat.

I wailed, "No. No. No." I burst into tears. I reached out to grasp someone and found the arms of the nurse, who hugged me until I had settled enough to call Bastian. I had to text him the news because I had no reception to make a call. Then I emailed my homeschool group for prayers.

It's a blur after this. All I remember is that I was still excited to meet baby Sloane. Everything in me longed for her. My husband arrived and was allowed to stay for twenty-four hours. I was induced, and the doctors opened my cervix with a balloon. In extreme discomfort, adrenaline racing, I waited for my baby to come.

She came easily because she only weighed around two pounds. She was small, but perfect. They put a cap on her and swaddled her and gave her to me. I couldn't cry, because she was so beautiful. I couldn't cry, because she looked alive. I couldn't cry, not yet, because I had her in my arms. I wiped a little bit of blood from the corner of her mouth. I opened her swaddle, and my Bastian and I held her little feet and hands.

When I was ready, Bastian swaddled her again and took her to the couch. I still have the image of her tiny body wrapped up safely in my husband's strong arms. When a nurse came for Sloane later, Bastian said with tears in his eyes, "How am I just supposed to hand her over? How am I supposed to just give her away?"

It made me think of our first baby, Ephesus Therese (Effie), who had died nine years earlier. She was our first life created together. Two and a half weeks after conception, we saw her little hands on the ultrasound, and then we were told she had died. That day, I learned to dread the moment between the start of an ultrasound and the first words spoken by the technician. I carried the remains of our Ephesus in my womb for thirty days after that ultrasound, waiting for my body to miscarry her, only to have a D&C. I hate that she was "removed" using a method abortionists use. We saw Effie once more on ultrasound before the brutal procedure, and how I prayed she would miraculously still be alive.

I never held Effie. When my husband offered me the tiny box of her remains at the church of burial, I refused. I wish I hadn't. I wish I would have felt the weight of her body in my hands. Now, Sloane's body was gone too. She was in a dark freezer somewhere in the basement of the hospital. The visions I had of her there are too terrible to share, but I didn't have time to dwell on them then, because my life was slowly draining away.

After vaginal labor, a nurse always presses on the abdomen to make sure everything has been delivered. My nurse kept coming back to push again. She pushed so hard, I threw my neck and shoulders out clenching the bed rails from the pain. I was bleeding out. Pools of blood were removed from the bed on giant plastic sheets. More nurses and doctors entered the room, and all their faces dropped. Everything went quiet. More blood was drawn, and infusions of platelets, cryo, and blood cells began. I heard a nurse in the hallway say, "We are out of blood. The Red Cross is flying some in."

I looked over at my husband who, following a nurse's suggestion, was asleep on the couch. I noticed five or six empty blood bags in the trash. I realized I was dying, and I got mad. "You took my child, and I wasn't mad at You, God, but now You want to take me too!? You can't do this to my children, to my husband. You cannot have me." I wrestled with God for a while, begging, pleading, denying Him my life.

I looked up at the TV screen on the wall, and a corny movie was on — *Groundhog Day*. It was the scene where a homeless man is dying, and Bill Murray tries to revive him. I couldn't believe what I was seeing.

A woman on the screen suddenly said, "Sometimes people just die." And Bill Murray responded triumphantly, "Not today!" I broke down. I felt God was answering. I knew I would live, but it didn't stop me from fearing death and seeing it in everything over the next few years. When will death strike again? Which of my children will it be? Why did you save me, Lord, and take my daughter instead? What purposes do you have for me? Are my purposes done? Will you take me now?

The doctors told me I had DIC — disseminated intravascular coagulation. It is a rare, life-threatening bodily response to trauma and is not well understood. For me, I suspect the trauma was the death of my baby in utero. The blood in the uterus clots after birth, and maybe my body thought I'd given birth, because the blood started clotting in my bloodstream. When I finally gave birth, I had no clotting agents left. When did you die, Sloane? How did I not notice you were gone?

After four days in the intensive care unit, I was moved back to the maternity ward. For two days, I heard newborns crying and families visiting the rooms around me. To cope, I started writing Sloane's life story in a journal my husband had dropped off. I imagined what she would have known of us through the sounds and sensations in the womb. I imagined Our Lady taking her to Heaven. This story is now a picture book called *Jellybean: A Baby's Journey to God*.

I never felt alone in the hospital. The nurses were truly sympathetic. One of them even found a rosary and put it in baby Sloane's hands for the memorial photos. Then she put it in the memorial box for me to take home. Hundreds of strangers and friends wrote to me online, sharing their stories of loss and the wisdom that only seasoned grievers have. They helped me find a free casket from the Trappist monks in Iowa, and they helped me find a funeral home with low rates for baby-sized plots. We raised over five thousand dollars in donations for the funeral and health expenses.

I left the hospital with a blood clot in my lung and a broken spirit. The night I came home, I lay in bed with my three-year-old daughter. Her pixie-like features and soft skin were like Sloane's. She seemed to sense my sorrow and threw her arms around me, nuzzling her head into mine. "Would Sloane have looked like you?" I thought.

My family had started a daily Rosary during the Covid lockdowns only a few months earlier. We prayed on video call while I was in the hospital. Once home, we came together every day, a little apprehensive, because we knew it would be painful to open our hearts. I cried at every Rosary for a long time, and my husband or one of my children usually joined me. My son would come give me small leg massages or my daughter would lay her head in my lap. Our bonds were strengthened, and we began to pray to our four children in Heaven. We decided to name the other two we had lost very early.

Each of my children suffered differently. My three-year-old asked a lot of questions, sometimes the same ones over and over. My son kept saying, "Why would I be sad when my sister got to go to Heaven?" For years, he was at peace, but the loss grieves him now. My oldest was nine when Sloane died. The funeral was surprisingly important for her. She sat in a chair next to the coffin, holding baby Sloane's hand for almost an hour. She didn't let go until the mortuary staff closed the lid, and then she placed a hand on the coffin all the way to the hearse.

She told me, "I was thinking that soon she would be under the ground forever, and I would never be able to see her again. So I decided that I would stay next to her the whole time."

My husband didn't really show emotions unless I pulled them out. He often said, "I am just too tired to be sad." But he noticed when I needed him. Once he saw me crying alone and said, "Get over here. You don't need to cry alone. I want you near me. I didn't think you were coming home."

Once I apologized for being "too needy," and he told me that he understood I was going to grieve harder than he did. He explained that my body was not only emotionally attached but also physically attached to Sloane. My hormones were telling me at a chemical level that something was always missing. The physical absence on top of the emotional anguish was the most painful part of my grief. I would just curl up in bed and ask Our Lady to hold me. "*When will this get easier?*" I wondered.

I was in shock for a while. I would suddenly remember that I had a baby and that she was dead, and I would choke. There was a beautiful path at the local community college, and I couldn't even look in its direction without being unable to breathe. It was the place I last remembered the baby kicking. I also felt like I couldn't breathe whenever I passed the baby section in Target. It took months to face my feelings and enter the ominous black holes that these two places had become.

My days at home were full of questions. I set to investigate the last days of my daughter's life, the places we visited, and the times I felt her movements. Did I kill you? If the platelet problems were a response to your death, how did you die? Did I gain too much weight? Did I do stretches that caused your cord to strangle you? Was I too stressed? Did I kill you by continuing anxiety medications, even though my doctor said I could?

Again, I remembered our first child, Effie. Weeks before she died in my womb, I created a mosaic flowerpot. My husband came home from work and said the house smelled toxic. I hadn't realized the glaze I was using was lingering in the air. The next few days, I was struck with a migraine so painful that I had to go to the ER for treatment. If the fumes made your mama that sick, what did they do to you, sweet Effie?

Then, there were the questions surrounding Heaven for unbaptized babies. Are my babies really in Heaven? Am I living a comforting lie when I pray to them? What do other Catholics think of me, especially when I share my belief with others at my Latin Mass parish that unbaptized babies go to Heaven? Do I push back when other moms tell me their babies are in the upper level of hell where they feel no pain but never receive the Beatific Vision? Do I take the time to engage in debate with my traditional and sympathetic priest about the problems with Limbo? Do I say I only "hope" in Heaven for my babies or is it alright to say I "believe" in it?

The day after the funeral, when I knew the only part of my baby I could touch was in the ground forever, the grief peaked. I felt I had lost her all over again. A few weeks later, I went to a retreat at my parish. At the beginning of Covid, the priests had erected a tent and a wooden altar, so Masses wouldn't have to be cancelled. Jesus was exposed in the Blessed Sacrament and incense gently swirled on a breeze.

I was meditating on a book called *Praying with Our Lady of Sorrows* by Eileen Tully, a mother who lost twins. I felt Our Lady had a hand on my shoulder, helping me face the grief. In the stillness, I began to break. So I prayed harder and held back my tears. Then a baby started to cry a few seats away. I wanted to snuggle and comfort him. The sorrow was crushing me. I wanted so badly to go weep in the front of the church alone with a statue of Our Lady of Guadalupe, but I felt bad leaving Jesus exposed on the altar.

Behind the altar hung a tapestry of Our Lady of the Angels by William-Adolphe Bouguereau. In it, Our Lady presents the Child Jesus to the world, surrounded by angels. I begged for solace and then glanced up at Our Lady. In an instant, I was struck! All at once, the image was alive, and Our Lady was holding my Sloane and floating toward me. She was holding Sloane with outstretched arms, and some deep part of me heard the words, "Look, I have her. It was I who gathered her up." I was immediately comforted. I felt permission from Christ to go weep at Mary's statue. Later, when I was interviewed by Christine Rossi on the radio show *A Light in the World*, she told me, "Where Jesus is, Our Lady cannot fail to be. They are always together."

The only way I can make sense of what I saw is to recall "Our Lady of the Smile." This is the title for Our Lady in a mystical experience St. Thérèse of Lisieux had. When Thérèse was young, she fell unexplainably ill. She hadn't been able to leave her bed for almost two months, so a statue of Our Lady was placed at her bedside. One day, she turned toward the statue to pray and saw Our Lady smile. This cured her! My moment of grace had come too, and my heart began to heal. This experience and reading the family letters of Sts. Louis and Zelie Martin in the book *Called to a Deeper Love* brought me lasting comfort.

Fear and grief still consume me sometimes, but I've learned to respond with prayer and surrender: "Your will be done, for You are always good, Lord." I'm now in the habit of pulling myself out of darkness with gratitude. I recall that I survived. I look back and see all the graces which prepared me for the loss of Sloane. I look at all the friends of loss I have made, how many people I have been able to help. I have so much to be grateful for! I've been given four children to guide us to Heaven and a profound connection with Our Blessed Mother.

Yet, a few questions still remain like scars on my heart. *Are you our last baby, Sloane? Will we ever have another? And … is it safe to?*

CHAPTER 16

Infant Loss

Twin A for Angel

Valerie Atkinson

My husband and I met in the fourth grade at Catholic grade school. Although we remained friends through high school and college, I never imagined that we would one day be married. As fate would have it, though, we started dating shortly after we both graduated and moved home from college — and the rest is history.

Even before we were married we had agreed that we wanted children, and two years into our marriage we were blessed with our oldest daughter, Catherine. We knew we wanted another child to complete our family and provide a sibling for Catherine; however, getting pregnant turned out to be harder the second time around. After more than a year of trying and more prayers than we could count, we were thrilled to find out we were pregnant with twins!

I had a very uneventful pregnancy, and at our twenty-week ultrasound found out we were expecting a girl and a boy. To say we were excited is an understatement. My husband and I finally agreed on names but decided to keep them a secret from our family and friends. Both babies continued to grow and look great at each ultrasound. Like many moms-to-be, I loved getting to see the babies at my appointments and watch in awe as they kicked, yawned, and wiggled around. The ultrasound techs always commented on what a full head of hair our baby girl had and how our little man was already causing trouble, kicking at his sister.

As my due date approached, we continued to prepare to welcome twins into our family. We already had a lot of baby things from our oldest, but of course now we needed two of everything! We purchased a second bouncer chair, high chair, car seat, and crib, as well as a bigger stroller. We turned our office into a nursery and began to fill it with all things baby. I spent my nights online, happily ordering clothes so the babies could have coordinating outfits, and carefully organizing them in their closet when they arrived. I remember standing in their room looking at everything and thinking, "*Wow, pretty soon two new babies will be using all of this stuff!*" It was overwhelming yet so exciting.

The ultrasound showed that baby A, our girl, was breech, and baby B, our little boy, was transverse, so I was scheduled for a C-section. Five days before my scheduled delivery, I began having contractions, so we went to the hospital early in the morning. I was thirty-seven weeks and five days along. As we got settled into our room it really hit me that today was the day we were going to meet our babies and become a family of five! We sat anxiously as doctors and nurses came in and out of the room and took a few last pictures of my now huge belly. For some odd reason, the only thing that worried me at the time was something happening to me during surgery that would leave my husband alone to raise three small children. Walking into the operating room was surreal. There were so many people there, including a team for each baby. I remember sitting on the operating table waiting for the anesthesiologist and seeing the warmers in front of me. One for baby A, the other for baby B. Never in my wildest dreams did I imagine I would be lucky enough to be in this position.

The incredible group of nurses calmed my nerves a bit, and once I was on the table waiting for the doctor I was finally at peace that things were going to be okay. At 12:46 p.m. on January 8, 2015, Elizabeth was born, followed by her brother, William, at 12:47 p.m. When the doctor announced that Elizabeth was out I immediately asked if she was okay, in my head thinking, "*Of course she is, but asking is just the thing to do.*" Elizabeth never cried. The doctors and nurses told my husband and me that she had just taken in some fluid and they needed to get it cleared out. Meanwhile, a screaming William was brought over to my side, which was a welcome distraction. As they wheeled me out of the operating room, I was able to get my first look at Elizabeth and touch her little hand. She was absolutely beautiful and, as predicted, came with a full head of dark hair.

Once we were settled in the recovery room, the nurses brought William in and we were told that Elizabeth had been brought to the NICU as she was still having trouble breathing. We were under the impression that she was fine and just needed to recover a bit from the delivery. The most shocking news of the afternoon was that Elizabeth weighed in at a whopping nine pounds, one ounce! With the addition of William's weight, six pounds, fifteen ounces, that meant I had been carrying sixteen pounds of baby. To this day I don't know how they fit!

That evening, we were able to visit Elizabeth in the NICU, as I still had not had a chance to hold her. When we got there, I was completely overwhelmed by all the tubes and monitors she was hooked up to. The nurse handed her to me, and I was so nervous that I would accidentally pull on something and hurt her. I just wanted to get her out of there and bring her back to my room, free of everything, but knew she needed to be there to get stronger. Two days later we got news that turned our world upside down. The NICU doctor informed us that he thought Elizabeth had a genetic disorder that was causing her not to be able to maintain her oxygen level and body temperature, but that they were still awaiting test results. There is nothing that can prepare you for the news that the beautiful baby you thought was perfectly healthy less than twenty-four hours ago is now suffering from a list of complications and that the doctors don't know why. I immediately broke down crying and started searching online about the list of disorders they were testing for. When we got the results of the first round of tests, we were relieved to find out they were all negative. While this was good news, it still left us wondering what was causing all the issues.

Three days after the twins were born, I faced another one of my biggest pregnancy fears, leaving the hospital with only one baby. Although I knew Elizabeth was in good hands, I absolutely hated leaving her behind. I was angry that we had prayed so hard for these babies and their health, and yet here we were. There were three other sets of twins born at the hospital on the same day as Elizabeth and William, and they all got to go home. Why weren't we that lucky?

The next few weeks were full of ups and downs as the NICU doctors continued to monitor and perform tests on Elizabeth. One day things would look good and she would be eating and completely off oxygen, and then we would get a phone call in the middle of the night that she had been put back on it. After four weeks in the NICU in our local hospital, we were told there was nothing more they could do, and we were given the option of bringing Elizabeth home on oxygen with a feeding tube or having her transferred to another hospital. As much as we wanted her home, we knew we needed to get to the bottom of her issues and decided to have her moved to a children's hospital two hours away. After many tense phone calls with our insurance company, the new hospital's transport team was finally given the go-ahead to come and get Elizabeth. It was an emotional day, leaving the doctors and nurses we had come to know so well and the familiar walls of the NICU, but also a day filled with hope that we were moving in the right direction toward getting Elizabeth healthy. We gave Elizabeth one last kiss and got in the car to meet her at the new hospital.

When we arrived, we got checked in at the Ronald McDonald House, which was across the street from the hospital — a blessing both in terms of proximity to Elizabeth and financially. That night, we met with Elizabeth's team and were told that within two weeks we would know if Elizabeth was improving or declining. As one can imagine, having a three-year-old and a newborn at home two hours away was not easy. I split my time between home and the children's hospital, while my husband stayed with Elizabeth. We had decided that it was better for him to stay with Elizabeth as he is the notetaker and remembered every detail the doctors and nurses said, while I was the emotional wreck who just wanted to hold my baby girl.

The days in the NICU were long, as our new team continued to run tests and monitor Elizabeth. One of the most memorable days was when we finally got to introduce our oldest daughter to her sister. She was not allowed in the NICU in our hometown, and we were so thankful that the new hospital allowed visitors under the age of eighteen. Catherine had waited so long to meet her sister, and it truly brought tears to our eyes to see her hold her for the first time.

Before we knew it, two weeks had passed and our care conference with Elizabeth's team of doctors was scheduled. I was at home the night before and had to make the drive back to the hospital that morning. In my heart I knew what they were going to tell us, as I had noticed Elizabeth getting weaker each time I saw her, but I just kept praying that I was wrong. When we entered the conference room, I immediately knew what they were going to tell us. Two of the people at the end of the table introduced themselves as members of the palliative care team. I knew what that meant. To be honest, I don't remember much more of what was said during the meeting. All I could hear were the silent screams in my head asking God why this was happening. We had so many people praying for our sweet Elizabeth, yet there was nothing more we or the doctors could do. She was continuing to decline, and they still had not found an exact diagnosis.

When we left the meeting, we made the decision to stop running tests on Elizabeth and just keep her as comfortable as possible. They had already tested for the things they could "fix," and my husband and I decided that having a name for what was wrong with her would not make us feel any more at peace with the situation. We were moved to a larger room where we could have a family visit and be with Elizabeth. For the first time since she was born, we could take her off all the monitors and hold her without the constant beeping of alarms. We had no idea how much time we had left with Elizabeth, whether it would be a few days or a few months.

On Valentine's Day, a day after our world had once again been turned upside down, we had Elizabeth baptized at the hospital. While it was not the picture-perfect day I had imagined of our twins being baptized together at our home parish, it was still a special day for all of us. We were also blessed to have a wonderful photographer from Now I Lay Me Down to Sleep come to the hospital and take pictures for us. This organization provides free portraits for families grieving the loss of an infant or stillbirth child. I didn't have any pictures of all three kids together or of our family at that point, so the images she captured are truly special to us.

All the doctors and nurses at the hospital were so wonderful and compassionate. In the craziness of processing that our daughter was dying, I never would have thought to get footprints, handprints, or make crafts, but the nurses did, and I am forever grateful to them. One person I will never forget was a member of the custodial team. I was alone in the room rocking Elizabeth when she came in to tidy up.

She saw my tears and stopped what she was doing. She smiled and said, "God's here, you know. It might not feel like it, but He's here." I never caught her name or saw her again, but what she said stuck with me. In that heartbreaking and awful moment sitting in that hospital room holding my dying baby girl, she said exactly what I needed to hear. Even at our worst moments we are never alone, God is always with us. This was a reminder I definitely needed.

For the next few days, I continued to go back and forth between the hospital and home. We were given the option of bringing Elizabeth home, but I just couldn't do it for some reason. I was afraid I wouldn't be able to handle watching her struggle at home without a doctor or nurse to call when there was an issue. It wasn't until I was in the shower at home one morning that I thought, "*What kind of mother doesn't let her daughter come home?*" God definitely spoke to me at that moment, and I knew where she needed to be. I immediately called my husband and told him I wanted her home. They quickly got the ball rolling, arranging her discharge and coordinating with hospice to come to our home. That evening, my husband and father-in-law brought Elizabeth home. We had no idea how long she would be with us, but it is a moment I will never forget. We finally had our family of five under one roof, even if only for a brief time. I was so mentally and physically exhausted that my dad offered to stay and spend the night holding Elizabeth.

The next morning, I got up and brought Catherine to preschool, as we were trying to keep her routine as normal as possible. When I got home, I had started to get ready for the day when my husband came into the bathroom and told me that Elizabeth did not look good. I ran to the living room and saw my sweet girl fading away. She had fought so hard and been through so much and I knew this was it. We called hospice and our families to come and be with us as we said goodbye to our baby girl. The priest from our parish came and prayed with us as I sat on the couch taking in every part of Elizabeth: her soft hair, her chubby cheeks, the way she kept her middle finger bent down, everything I didn't want to ever forget. The hospice nurse kept coming over to check on Elizabeth, and each time I prayed that we would have a little bit longer with her. Then came the moment we knew was coming but could never have been prepared for. The nurse came to listen to her heartbeat and there wasn't one. Our baby girl was gone from this earth.

While many tears were shed at that moment, it was also a moment of peace, knowing that Elizabeth was free of all her earthly struggles. We knew without a doubt that she was in Heaven and that we would see her again someday. Elizabeth was five weeks and six days old when she died on February 18, 2015, which was Ash Wednesday. When we receive ashes, the priest speaks the words, "Remember that you are dust and to dust you shall return." This rang especially true on this day and has every Ash Wednesday since Elizabeth's passing.

The next few days were spent planning Elizabeth's funeral Mass, picking out flowers, and making arrangements at the cemetery. I remember walking through the store with tears in my eyes, trying to find something for William to wear to the funeral. It was all a blur. Knowing I had to stay strong for Catherine and William is what got me out of bed in the morning. While Catherine was only three at the time, she was keenly aware of what was going on. It was a struggle to find the right words to explain things to her, and I honestly don't know what we would have done without our faith. Since Elizabeth was born we had explained to her that God makes each of us different and special in our own way. We told her that Elizabeth was not born strong like she and William were and that she was going to go to Heaven to be with Jesus. I was always afraid that if we said that Elizabeth was "sick," Catherine would be terrified that she or one of us would die too from a simple cold. Although Catherine was upset that she couldn't have her sister at home with us, she was very understanding and okay with the idea that she would be an angel in Heaven watching over us.

Elizabeth's funeral was held on a Saturday morning. We referred to it as her "special Mass," as that seemed to go over better with Catherine. It was overwhelming to see Elizabeth in her little white casket, looking as beautiful as ever. It was also overwhelming to see all the people who came to support our family. It meant so much to be with our family and friends and hear stories from others who had lost children at all different stages of life. Seeing everyone who came made me understand why you should "go to the funeral." If not for the person who died, go for those who have been left behind.

The Mass was beautiful and a moment when God truly felt present. As we walked out of the church and said our final goodbyes, the words of one of the songs we had chosen, "Go in Peace," stuck in my head. "Lift your heart, rejoice and sing for you are home. Home at last and forever in the arms of the holy one." The phrase "You are home" is still with me today. As sad as it was to say goodbye to our sweet girl, she was in her forever home — a place we can all only hope and pray to one day be.

The days and weeks that followed were tough. We had gone from the craziness of going back and forth between the hospital and home for almost six weeks to what seemed like an awkward stillness. We were left to clear out a nursery full of things for two babies and find a way to go on with life down a completely different path than we had imagined. My husband and I were extremely aware of the divorce statistics for couples who had lost a child and knew that no matter what, we had to find a way to stay together for us and our other children. We each grieved in our own way, but our faith in God was our constant. We continued to go to Mass each week and to pray every day. While there were and still are difficult moments, we found a way to get through them. For me, I liked talking about Elizabeth and hearing others' stories, so I decided to attend a SHARE meeting at the hospital where the twins were born.

While driving to my first meeting, I panicked and thought that maybe I shouldn't go, that I was fine and didn't need to talk to anyone about it. However, Elizabeth was there with me and gave me a sign. In the middle of a completely sunny evening, there was a rainbow in front of me as I got on the highway. I ended up going and found the group of people there to be a true blessing. I enjoyed the support of those who had walked a similar path and found inspiration in the things they had done to heal their hearts and honor the children they had lost.

My husband didn't feel the need to attend meetings to get him through. He had spent the most time of all of us with Elizabeth and I know they had something special. To this day, he still talks to her on his drive to work in the morning. While we seemed to be doing well as a couple considering the circumstances, one of our biggest disagreements was about the idea of another child. We had agreed that our family would be complete with the addition of the twins, but in my mind everything changed when Elizabeth died. I didn't feel like that was how our story was supposed to end, and I believed God had plans for our family to grow. My husband, on the other hand, was happy with the children we had already been blessed with and was hesitant to try again after everything we had been through. We agreed that the idea was not completely off the table and we would take a "let go and let God" approach.

Shortly after the twins turned one, we got the surprise of a lifetime. I was pregnant! I thought for sure this was God's way of helping us heal, a rainbow baby to complete our family. I took cute pictures of William holding a big brother sign and showed my parents. Everyone was thrilled by the news. Almost as quickly as we celebrated, however, we all came crashing down.

Less than a week after we found out I was pregnant, my doctor's office called with the news that my HCG levels had dropped and that I was losing the baby. I was heartbroken. I just kept thinking, "*How could God do this to our family again?*" We prayed, went to church, worked hard to live and raise our children in a faith-filled way. I thought to myself, "*That's it. We are done going to church!*" This moment was probably the truest test of my faith that I have experienced so far. As much as I wanted to be mad at God and throw in the towel, I knew I couldn't. Our faith in God is what got our family through and continues to sustain us after losing Elizabeth. The thought of leaving our church community and the Catholic school that meant so much to us was more than I could handle. This was just another moment when we needed to pray to persevere and a reminder that God walks beside us in the good and the bad. I had started listening to Christian radio, and a song that really spoke to me in yet another difficult time was "Hills and Valleys" by Torin Wells. The words of the song are so true. God is with us in the good and the bad and we are never, ever alone. Just have faith.

After the miscarriage, I was forced to come to grips with the fact that maybe our family was complete. I was not happy about it, but once again trusted that God had a plan for us. Two years later His plan became clear. I became pregnant again, and my due date was February 16, two days before Elizabeth died. While we were thrilled with the news, I was absolutely terrified. There were several scares throughout my pregnancy, but I prayed harder than I had ever prayed before. As a way to try to calm my nerves, I saw my doctor every week and found a few short Bible passages I read before every appointment. One of my favorites that I still read is Psalm 112:7 (NRSVCE): "They are not afraid of evil tidings; their hearts are firm, secure in the LORD." I was so afraid of what might happen at each appointment; it was helpful to read this passage over and over and remind myself not to be afraid and to once again have confidence in God.

During the many long nights when I couldn't sleep, I would grab the rosary off my nightstand and pray. On February 12, 2019, our daughter Jean was born. While she in no way replaces Elizabeth, she has brought so much joy to our lives and I finally have a sense that our family is complete. The constant wondering "*Will this be the month I get pregnant*?" was over, and my mind was at peace. God truly does work in mysterious ways.

While our story may not be picture-perfect, it is ours. We are so very blessed by what God has given us and definitely stronger and more faith-filled people because of the obstacles we have faced along our journey. The struggles we have been through have tested our faith but have also helped it to flourish. We have gained the friendship of so many people who have lost children, and we have definitely become more compassionate toward others. It has made us truly appreciate every single day that God gives us and makes me slow down and cherish the moments I get with my children. I still pray for the baby we lost to miscarriage, and we include Elizabeth in everything we do. We celebrate her birthday as if she were here on earth, with a cake and singing, and remember her on the anniversary of her death, which we call her "angelversary." We find joy in decorating her headstone at the cemetery for every holiday and season and talk about what we think she would be like today. Each fall we do a remembrance walk with the SHARE group in her honor, and we have a framed picture of her that one of us always holds in our family photos to be sure she is included.

One of my biggest fears has always been that Elizabeth will be forgotten, so it is my personal mission to make sure she is not. It means so much when people mention her name or ask how we are doing. Even though it has been four years, it still seems like yesterday. While we have come a long way, we will never be the same. I saw a blog from a mom who described life after child loss as living on the edge of tears, and I couldn't agree more. Whether it is a song, or what should be a first day of school, or hearing her name, I feel as though I am vulnerable to a breakdown at any moment. On the good days and bad, I remember to put my trust in God. He has a plan for each of us, and though we might not fully understand it yet, we need to have faith. Although I know there will be hills and valleys ahead for our family, I am confident that our faith will get us through and that we always have God by our side.

CHAPTER 17

Infant Loss

Luke's Story

Taylor and Melissa Blanton

Melissa: March 11, 2017, 3 a.m. Something just didn't feel right. I immediately took a pregnancy test. I let Taylor sleep for about four more hours before I started poking him in the shoulder. "Hey! Hey! Are you awake? I think I'm pregnant." A second pregnancy test had the same result, and ten days later blood tests made it official. We were pregnant! Although Taylor wanted to wait a little longer, I couldn't keep it in anymore (it is hard to hide nausea and morning sickness), so we told our parents on March 26. An ultrasound on March 29 gave us our first glimpse at "#babybleezy," and we first heard the heartbeat! We were so excited! Next came our first appointment with my doctor, which was in mid-May, and we scheduled our ultrasound for June.

As we ended the first trimester, we started to go public: #baby bleezy is joining our pack! Friends and family heard the good news. Family members sent me gifts, and Taylor's coworkers danced with him. On June 8, I was scheduled to go in late for work, and Taylor was going to head straight to school for the first day of his summer class after our appointment. We were anxious to find out whether we were having a boy or a girl. We would be overjoyed either way, but when we found out it was a boy, we were over the moon.

The ultrasound technician, though, was using carefully selected words, not fully answering our questions, and the mood in the room quickly changed. She spent a long time looking at certain things on that grainy black-and-white screen. As she left the room, she said, "The doctor will be in shortly with some very serious things to discuss."

After the doctor joined us, did another ultrasound, and began to hint at some complications, Taylor and I canceled our work days. I wouldn't see patients in my optometry practice, and Taylor, a teacher, would not be there for his first day of class. After an hour of images, discussions, and consultations with the doctors, we were heartbroken. Right hypoplastic heart syndrome. No pulmonary artery. Enlarged heart. No room for the lungs to develop. Soft markers for chromosomal abnormalities. (An echocardiogram with a pediatric cardiologist on July 6 confirmed all of the above, as well as two additional problems with the baby's heart valves.)

After spending most of the day at the hospital, we returned home. We asked both sets of parents to come over to the house, where we told them what we knew at that point. They told the rest of our immediate family, but we kept things private for the time being. We wanted to get away and spend some time together, so we decided to go to Wilmington the next day for a beach weekend. Wrightsville Beach, a walk at Airlie Gardens, Mass at St. Mark's Church, and dinner in downtown Wilmington. We slept in Sunday morning, went back to the beach again, then headed home, back to real life.

During the weekend, Taylor and I had some serious discussions about our son and our path forward. First of all, we knew our faith and trust were in God and His plan, period. As challenging as the thought was (and still is), our baby boy was always God's child first and ours second. From the moment his life began, he was our son, and therefore he needed a name. We considered many options, but we kept coming back to two names. Taylor suggested one, and I brought up the other. We loved the names, and the reason behind them: Luke Michael, the physician apostle and the archangel fighter who leads God's army into battle.

On Father's Day, Sunday, June 18, we went to evening Mass at our home parish, the church where Taylor and I were married. Father Steve, the officiant at our wedding, was presiding over Mass that evening. Afterward, our parents joined us as I received the sacrament of the Anointing of the Sick. It was there that we first told our parents, and Father Steve, that our baby boy's name was Luke Michael. This brought an extra smile to my dad's (Michael's) face. In the weeks that followed, we slowly began letting people know. It was usually after someone asked how we were doing, or how I was feeling. We never meant to hide anything from anyone, but it wasn't something we wanted to bring up.

As we progressed through the pregnancy, many thoughts crossed our minds. Although we had no idea what the future held, we strongly believed that as long as Luke had a pulse, he had a purpose, and we planned to do everything in our power to help him achieve that purpose.

Taylor: Melissa and I were married for just over a year before we got pregnant. It was a beautiful ceremony, a great reception with our friends and family, and our first year of marriage was wonderful. It was amazing to me how quickly it felt normal, as if we had always been married. Preparing for the actual wedding, though, was a different story. Picking out the napkin colors, the food choices, and all the rest can be overwhelming. What made it even more stressful for us was that we tend to be very private people. We don't like to be the center of attention, and everything about the event put us in the center. Although that is obviously the entire point, we were looking forward more to the marriage than the wedding itself!

Now we found ourselves here, thirteen months later, sharing our very private lives with everyone again. We knew that our journey with Luke would have many challenges, and to be honest, living this part of our lives publicly was one of those challenges. But we knew that it was also a great blessing. God blessed Melissa and me in so many ways during that time, and continues to do so. Our parents, sisters, grandparents, and extended family supported us; our priests, ministers, and Sunday-school teachers have taught and counseled us; our friends have shared awesome memories and have been with us through thick and thin. In this season of life, we knew that these were the people God had put in our lives to help us.

After we found out we were pregnant, we wondered when we would find out whether it was a boy or a girl. Melissa was more inclined to be surprised at birth, but I, the meticulous planner, wanted to know as soon as possible. Lucky for me, I brought her over to my side. We also talked about whether we preferred a girl or a boy. Perhaps it was the fact that we had recently started watching *Last Man Standing* on Netflix, but I had images in my mind of being overwhelmed in a house full of women. I (not so) secretly was pulling for a boy! I remember one morning in the first trimester. Melissa and I were still lying in bed when we started praying aloud. We prayed for guidance and wisdom, and for us to follow God's will, "but if there happens to be flexibility on the will, I'd really like a boy!" I added. At this, Melissa busted out laughing, but I think she agreed with my sentiments. We were so happy that God answered our prayer to be Luke's parents!

Since that point, we had met with more doctors, nurses, and specialists than I can remember. Hypoplastic right heart syndrome is a condition in which the right side of the heart is significantly underdeveloped. It is the right ventricle that pumps blood to the lungs, and combined with the additional problems with the valves in Luke's heart, this presented a serious challenge. Hypoplastic left heart syndrome occurs in approximately one in five thousand newborns, but hypoplastic right heart syndrome is much rarer. There are two treatment methods for the disease: a three-stage surgical procedure (surgery at approximately seven days, at six months, and at two to five years old), or a heart transplant. Both of these entail significant risk, but Luke had several obstacles he would need to overcome before one of these surgeries was possible.

As a result of the underdeveloped right side of the heart, his left side was doing extra work, causing it to grow significantly larger than it should. A baby's heart should occupy about one-third of the chest cavity. Luke's heart was taking up about 80 percent of the space. This prevented there being enough room for the other organs to grow and develop — most significantly, the lungs. Luke's lung growth and development was what we mainly prayed for throughout the pregnancy.

On a normal, daily basis, without the knowledge we had been given by the doctors and the tests they had run, it felt like a normal pregnancy. While Melissa had a tougher first trimester, she felt much better during the second. Luke liked to make his presence known with a good kick now and then. He liked to move around a lot, especially when we were trying to get a good look at him during the ultrasounds!

Earlier on in the diagnostic process, we sometimes marveled at how short periods of time felt like an eternity. In the struggles (and yes, we had moments where it was quite a struggle), we were constantly reminded of the blessings we have. When we feel empty and motionless, God is the wind in our sails. When we feel tossed about, He is our anchor in the waves. We trusted what God had in store for us. He gave us Luke, and we got to be his advocates and to fight for and with him. We had wonderful people who were with us on this journey.

The remaining months of the pregnancy were a long four months, but we persevered. Besides, I am a huge *Star Wars* fan. I couldn't wait to say, "Luke, I am your father!"

Melissa: "I felt that! Was that it?" I nodded. Taylor put his hand back on my stomach and waited. A few seconds later: "I felt it again! Was that it too?" I smiled and nodded again. While I had been feeling Luke tossing and turning and kicking up a storm for a few weeks, mid- to late July was the first time that Taylor could feel him. It was a high mixed in with the lows we had been experiencing. Although his movements were encouraging, they also made me feel like I was on a roller coaster, reminiscent of the first-trimester nausea, but it was also a roller coaster of emotions.

Following an echocardiogram (that seemed to take forever) with the pediatric cardiologist on July 27, we had a good but difficult conversation with the doctor. We knew that Luke had a tough diagnosis. Despite some doctors and nurses attempting to be sensitive to our situation, we were able to put two and two together, and we understood that our chances of spending more than a few moments with Luke, or even getting to meet him, were quite slim. On this day, though, that information was confirmed. It was incredibly difficult, heart-wrenching, and painful to hear, but we knew we were already on the path toward a peace that only God could provide. Although nothing was certain, we continued to believe in and hope for a miracle. We trusted whatever God had in store for us.

As long as Luke was in utero, he was safe and growing, and we continued to pray for his healing and his lung growth. As we had additional discussions with the doctors, we believed that a heart transplant, not the three-phase surgery procedure, would give Luke the best chance for a positive outcome. But we had many hurdles to get over before then.

In August, Taylor began his eleventh year as a teacher. It was surreal at times how life continued on as normal, even as our world had been irrevocably altered. Taylor and I tried to be more intentional with our time. Maybe a little more spontaneous, too, especially with date nights and weekend road trips. We visited Monticello. We traveled to the mountains to revisit the spot where we got engaged in May 2015.

We transferred Luke to another hospital to get him the best care possible. It was a decision I agonized over, but I remembered that in the end I am not in control. I trusted that God would guide the doctors and nurses just as He guided our decisions. We met with a neonatologist and a high-risk perinatal clinical nurse. Discussions about palliative care started, although we continued to hope and pray that Luke would prove everyone wrong! We felt supported and heard at our hospital of choice. We also found great support working with a perinatal hospice program, Be Not Afraid (www.benotafraid.net), and a birth and bereavement doula, Angela.

I loved feeling him move on a daily basis. At Monticello, Luke seemed extra active. Taylor said it is because he liked Thomas Jefferson — just like his daddy! He started to respond to Taylor's voice and move when Taylor talked to him. Such precious memories. Part of me wanted to stay pregnant forever so we could keep him safe and healthy. I often reflected on and tried to draw strength from Mary's life and her yes to God. There were many nights of tears, and I hated not knowing how this story would end.

I lectored at Mass for the feast of the Assumption of Mary. One of the Prayers of the Faithful I read to the congregation was: "For all mothers, that they find the strength to fulfill their vocation." This was difficult to hear, and especially to say, but I held it together. God always found big and small ways to constantly remind us that, however difficult, we were never alone in this journey.

As we entered the third trimester, Luke's heart continued to grow, occupying most of his chest cavity. At this point, we were told his lungs were likely too small to support life. However, we were over the moon to hear that the doctors did not think there were any other issues! We were so blessed to have an amazing ultrasound technician who sent us home with lots of pictures of his precious face. Although medically unlikely, we were also reassured by the neonatologist that there was still time for "things to change." So we continued to pray that his lungs would grow.

Taylor: Labor Day weekend provided a wonderful break from work for Melissa and me, three days of relaxing at home and seeing family and friends. It was also a respite from the visits to the doctor — two the week before and one upcoming during Labor Day week. While we were happy with our hospital of choice and the support we received there, it was still difficult to go through the rounds each time we made our way to the hospital.

While it appeared that Luke did not have any other genetic or growth abnormalities, his heart condition and limited lung growth remained a steep mountain to climb. Our pediatric cardiologist had sent Luke's information to the medical schools at the University of California at San Francisco and the University of Michigan, as well as to Boston Children's Hospital. All the doctors who reviewed his file agreed with his prognosis, and none of them had seen a heart quite like Luke's. The plan continued to be a heart transplant, if Luke's lungs were functional and if he could survive long enough to be stable. Unfortunately, that still appeared unlikely. Despite the uncertainty, with our due date in just over two months, we were excited to finally meet little Luke!

Melissa: "Life isn't fair" crossed my mind more times than I would like to admit during pregnancy. Too often, I would be jealous of other women's "normal" pregnancies ... the gender-reveal parties ... the baby showers … the glowing baby-bump pictures. And to be honest, this is still a struggle. But after reading Matthew 20:1–16 one weekend in September, and being reminded of one of my favorite musicals, *Joseph and the Amazing Technicolor Dreamcoat,* I was convicted. I could grumble like the laborers in the Gospel, but in reality, I didn't understand God's plan. We cannot see the larger picture. God is orchestrating a million moving parts in the overall plan of our lives, and our view is too narrow. "For my thoughts are not your thoughts, neither are your ways my ways, says the LORD" (Isa. 55:8). In Genesis chapters 37–50, Joseph had several "life isn't fair" moments. He was sold into slavery by his brothers as a teen, after being his father's favorite child. Then, just as he's back on top as Potiphar's servant, Potiphar's wife falsely accuses him and he lands in jail. Finally, he catches a break when Pharaoh needs a dream interpreter. If you don't know the rest of the story, Joseph reunited with his brothers some twenty-three years later. God needed Joseph in Pharaoh's service at that moment in time to save his family from starvation. The big picture took twenty-three years to take shape. There was purpose in Joseph's pain and struggles. God had not abandoned him. What an incredible reminder that our story wasn't anywhere near the end, and God was always with us!

At thirty-four weeks, we were stable. God is good, all the time! We wrote a birth plan and packed my hospital bag. We met with a volunteer photographer who would help document Luke's birthday. A friend gifted us with a beautiful maternity photography session. At our third appointment with our pediatric cardiologist, he could see blood flow in and out of Luke's lungs! He noted that this information should be neither more positive nor more negative than previous findings, but that he "hoped Luke would give us the chance to treat him." Our son's lungs continued to be the limiting factor, and we continued to pray. We knew his lungs would need every last day of the pregnancy to grow, so we hoped to avoid an early labor.

With one month left in the pregnancy, I experienced every emotion possible: fear, excitement, dread, elation, anxiety, and hope. Taylor and I had found a new normal in the "limbo" in which we lived. While not always the most pleasant, we had found peace and comfort in the unknown. We were now standing on the cusp of "the future." Although I have previously said I'd have loved to stay pregnant forever if it meant keeping Luke healthy and alive, that was not a possibility. It was time to take another leap of faith, and trust that God would be there to catch us. We continued to pray that Taylor and I remain steadfast in our hope, and would remember to place our trust *completely* in God's hands.

Taylor: At just over five months since we found out about Luke's diagnosis, we had found our "new normal." During that time, there were regular visits to doctors and the hospital, research and planning, and lots and lots of praying. We walked the line of trying to decide who and when to tell, all the while trying not to let it consume our daily lives. Now we found ourselves at the end of this journey and ready to see what God had in store for us next.

Luke was due any day now. His diagnosis had not changed. His heart complications were severe and would require a full heart transplant very soon after birth. As we knew, however, his enlarged heart had prevented other organs from being able to grow, including the lungs. When he arrived, he would be taken immediately to the NICU, where doctors would test his lungs. If they were functional, they would attempt to stabilize him and try to get him on a donor list. Obviously, finding a suitable match for a newborn, and then the operation itself, were also significant challenges. (Not to mention the conflicting emotions surrounding how a match would be found.) However, the more likely scenario was that the lung tests would reveal little functionality. This would indicate that Luke would be with us for a very short time, and we would then spend that time together as a family for as long as we had.

Melissa: We checked into the hospital early on the morning of November 15, 2017. As Luke had not arrived on his own, the plan was to induce labor. I was well supported by Taylor; my best friend, Jen; and my doula, Angela, during labor. Luke Michael was born at approximately 4:25 a.m. on November 16. His daddy baptized him immediately. He gave one little squeak of a cry, which brought tears of joy and a "Praise God!" from me. He was immediately taken to the NICU.

Taylor: Luke was termed "critically stable" when he was admitted to the NICU. He made some noises and cries at birth, which was a joy to hear considering our concerns about his lungs. He was immediately intubated in an effort to help him stabilize and prepare for the next challenge, extubation, to see if he could breathe on his own. In the first thirty hours of life, he proved himself to be a fighter and worthy of his name. He remained in the NICU, where the doctors and nurses watched him constantly. He was hooked up to so many things — it was both joyful and difficult to see him.

After Melissa was discharged, we made two to three trips a day to see Luke. We cherished the days when his eyes were open and he would wrap his tiny hands around our fingers. The first attempt to extubate Luke was beautiful. At first, he was mad — but I guess any of us would be if we had a tube taken out of our throat and lungs! He was crying quietly, making occasional sounds. His grandparents went in and saw him too. He had calmed down remarkably after about thirty minutes. He even gave a semi-smile back to us!

Melissa: We were told that our journey in the NICU would be like a dance — two steps forward, three steps back. We celebrated the milestones and the small victories when they happened (like changing Luke's diaper for the first time!). After extubation, the plan was to place Luke's peripherally inserted central catheter (PICC) line. Unfortunately, that was unsuccessful. In the stress, Luke struggled to remove the carbon dioxide from his body. So he was reintubated. We knew this could happen, and although we were disappointed, we continued to hope they would try to extubate him again soon.

I held Luke for the first time on Thanksgiving Day. I believe that experience was probably the closest I will get to Heaven here on earth: Watching the monitors with his heart rate and breathing rate sync with mine. Feeling him relax in my arms. His incredibly soft skin. What beautiful memories. The day after Thanksgiving was Taylor's turn to hold Luke. Be still, my new mama's heart. I am not sure there is anything sweeter than watching the man you love hold your new baby.

After Taylor went back to work I would spend a good portion of my day at Luke's bedside. We had lots of visitors while in the NICU, including a chaplain, an ICN parent care coordinator, and a physical therapist. During the assessment with the physical therapist, she said that Taylor looked familiar. (We had a picture of us taped up in Luke's bay.) I mentioned where he teaches and that seemed to be the connection. However, a couple of minutes later, her eyes widened and she said, "Wait, is this Luke? *The* Luke that the school community has been praying for?" All I could do was nod with tears in my eyes. This little man was so very loved by so very many people! I do not believe in coincidences. Coincidences are small miracles or "God sightings" in our lives. (I cannot take credit for coining the term.) Meeting this wonderful PT was my God sighting for that day. Our God continued to show us that He had Luke in the palm of His hands.

The second extubation attempt did not go well, and Luke struggled. It took him several days to recover. During that same week, our awesome PT taught me how to massage Luke's feet in an effort to give him some "good touch." Luke seemed to enjoy it, and I definitely loved any opportunity to connect with my little man. The times that Luke and I could do skin-to-skin holding were my favorite. There are no words to describe the amazing feeling of listening to your almost three-week-old baby's heart beat with yours.

Taylor had some profound words that stayed with me during our NICU time. We had so many people praying for Luke's healing, and maybe we were looking for a big miracle, but in reality his life was a series of small miracles. Our God is extraordinary. We continued to hope and pray that the small miracles would continue — each one taking us one step closer to taking our son home.

Luke continued to show his fighting spirit. He even self-extubated at one point! Our cardiology, neonatology, and cardiothoracic surgeons consulted with each other and with CHOP and Boston to discuss Luke's unique case. After another extubation attempt, Luke's body began to show fatigue. Taylor and I had consistently said that we wanted to prolong life, not suffering, in our attempt to save our son. After discussions with our team, it was decided that Luke was beyond the help of modern medicine. We would wean Luke off his oxygen, extubate him, make him comfortable, and let him go home to God. Fr. Daniel gave Luke the sacraments of Anointing of the Sick and Confirmation the day before his last.

The medical team expected we would have a couple of hours with Luke after he was extubated. Miraculously, we were blessed with more than eight hours before Luke went home to his Heavenly Father. Eight hours of cuddles and skin-to-skin. We sang and read books. We told stories about funny dates that Taylor and I went on. We laughed and we cried. My biggest fear was being traumatized by Luke's death. At the end, though, Luke was calm and peaceful. He took his last breath in my arms, with Taylor next to me rubbing his back. We were surrounded by his grandparents, aunts, and uncles. His death was truly a holy moment, and everyone in the room felt it. I wish I had the words to describe it more accurately. Although our hearts were broken, we know that we were not alone on this journey.

There are those who have gone before us, and many who continue to walk with us now. Grief changes you forever.

My very brave, amazing husband shared these thoughts at Luke's funeral:

> Thank you everyone for being here today.
>
> This part of our journey began when we found out about Luke's diagnosis in June 2017, and since then, we have been so incredibly loved and supported. The number of people who have supported us through prayers, meals, gifts, time, and so many other ways are countless, and you helped Melissa and me more than you will know. It wasn't easy, but I wanted to share a few moments that we experienced along the way.
>
> One day over the summer, a package arrived for us at our home. When we opened it, we found a beautiful blanket with Luke Michael embroidered on it, as well as "Precious in his sight," referring to the verse Jeremiah 1:5. That blanket covered Luke almost every day of his life. Other blankets, socks, and beanies were given, and they all mean so very much to us. Thank you.
>
> On a retreat with a group of my senior students in October, I shared with some students for the first time about Luke's diagnosis. Afterward, a student and cross-country runner came over to me and shared that every male member of his family had the middle name Michael, and that every one of them have a St. Michael medal. He then gave me his medal. That medal hung by my bed until Luke arrived, and it hung over Luke every day of his life.
>
> During the pregnancy, we had no idea whether or not we would be able to meet Luke. We did everything in our

power, including the incredible strength and bravery of my wife during labor, to ensure that we gave Luke the best chance to make it here. He did, and we were blessed with thirty-one days of life with him.

In very difficult and trying times like this, we can doubt and question our faith. To all my brothers and sisters in Christ, please know that our God is good.

Isaiah 57:1–2 says, "The righteous perish … the devout are taken away, and no one understands that the righteous are taken away to be spared from evil. Those who walk uprightly enter into peace; they find rest." Luke was spared any more discomfort, any more pain. While Melissa and I truly rejoice in that fact, it is still a terrible burden that we must carry.

Matthew 11:28–30 says, "Come to me, all you who are weary and burdened, and I will give you rest. Take my yoke upon you and learn from me, for I am gentle and humble in heart, and you will find rest for your souls. For my yoke is easy and my burden is light." Even in this immediate aftermath, Melissa and I have had brief moments of complete peace. Please pray for us that God would grant Melissa and me rest and peace as we move forward.

For all my brothers and sisters in Christ, we know that our time on this earth is just a brief moment compared to the eternity that awaits us afterward. A few months ago, Melissa and I were at church singing "Oh Come to the Altar." One of the lines is "Oh come to the altar, the Father's arms are open wide." During that song, I had a distinct image or vision in my mind. I saw a little boy from behind, walking into the presence of God. John 14:2, our Gospel reading for today, says, "My Father's house has many rooms; if that were not so, would I have told you that I am going there to prepare a place for you?" We know that Luke is with his Heavenly Father, even as his earthly father and mother miss him terribly.

Also at church recently, we were watching a video of another family, and in it, we were reminded that the purpose of life is to advance the Kingdom of God. Luke's life did that. He brought so many people together. He inspired so many people. He had prayers lifted up for him from Pennsylvania, Illinois, Florida, Arizona, California, Great Britain, the Netherlands, and Australia, among many other places. His impact was global.

I want to thank my parents, Melissa's parents, our sisters and brothers, for being with us over the past several days. They provided comfort to Luke, but also comfort to Melissa and me. We spent time together, with Luke, holding him, singing songs, and reading stories. We also told family stories and moments from the time Melissa and I met each other through our engagement. One special moment was me holding Luke, my father next to me, and my grandfather next to him. Four generations of Blanton men together. We were the twelfth, thirteenth, fourteenth, and fifteenth generations of Blanton men in America, three hundred and seventy years after Thomas Blanton came from England to Virginia in 1647.

We read *The Very Bumpy Bus Ride, Henry's Awful Mistake,* and *But No Elephants,* among others. These were some of my favorite books growing up that my parents read to me. We also read Luke a children's picture Bible from cover to cover, so he knew every Bible story.

We sang songs as well. "The Itsy Bitsy Spider," "Twinkle Twinkle Little Star," "The NC State Fight Song," the Presidents song, and I may have hummed the John Adams theme song too. We covered all of the important things. But the songs we sang most often were "Jesus Loves Me, This I Know" and "Jesus Loves the Little Children."

One song we sang as we were preparing to say goodbye is a Christmas song, but going forward, in my mind, it will be Luke's song. It is a song about Jesus, but other than Jesus' miraculous conception, it so perfectly captured everything about that moment.

Silent Night, holy night
All is calm, all is bright.
Round yon virgin, mother and child.
Holy Infant, so tender and mild.
Sleep in heavenly peace, Sleep in heavenly peace.

Sleep in heavenly peace, Luke. Mommy and Daddy love you forever.

Part III

PRACTICAL WISDOM

CHAPTER 18

For the Grieving Heart

The time following the loss of a baby is numbing and painful as you try to navigate all of the emotions that are flooding your entire being. The grieving process is complex and leaves you wondering when your heart will find healing again, when normalcy will return to your life.

Perhaps you and your spouse were the only ones who knew about the pregnancy, which may further the feelings of loneliness as you try to cope with this on your own. You attempt to put on a smile when you leave the house, but the reality is, you are broken.

It is important to give yourself time, acknowledge that this was indeed a loss no matter how far along you were, and give yourself permission to grieve. The following are practical steps and things to remember that may help with the grieving process.

Pray: On the hard days, prayer may be the last thing you want to do as you wrestle with frustration and anger toward God. It may even feel as if God has abandoned you. Having a child is such a noble and good intention, why would He deny you this gift? God is with you in the silence. He is carrying you through the valley. He is pouring out His grace and mercy and only wants you to rest in His arms as He heals your broken heart.

It may be difficult to formulate any words, but you can turn to the rote prayers. Pray with your husband for healing and ask him to speak the words when you cannot. It may seem simple, but there is great power in repeating the name of Jesus. Jesus, I trust in You! Keep praying the novenas and let your fingers run over the rosary beads. Ask others to pray for you, especially your spouse, your family, your friends, and your parish community. Sit in Eucharistic Adoration and say nothing at all. Go on a silent retreat and let God do the talking.

Honor: This child was real, a created being, not just tissue or the product of conception. A baby, your baby. Name your child even if you are not sure of the gender; choose something meaningful to you. Your little one is now with our Heavenly Father gazing upon His glory, so call upon him or her to intercede for you.

Have a memorial or a burial service. Call your pastor to see if he can have a small prayer service with you and your spouse or pray the blessing after a miscarriage with you. If a procedure was done, request the remains from the hospital. Organizations such as Elizabeth Ministry offer small burial vessels.

Remember: Do something to remember your child; it can be simple, such as a bouquet of flowers on the anniversary of his or her passing, or a balloon release with your family, attaching love notes to your little one. You could also have something personalized, such as a remembrance ring or bracelet, or birthstone for their anniversary month.

At age-appropriate levels talk about the baby with your other children; they are part of your family and a sibling to this child. Create a scrapbook for children ages one to ten who have died, so that older and future siblings can remember them.

Journal: What was wrong with me? Why am I inadequate? What if my spouse blames me? Will he love me less? The questions running through your mind may seem unreasonable at times, but allow yourself to feel what you are truly feeling.

It is normal to let your mind give way to unreasonable thoughts. Writing down the thoughts and feelings that are hard to express can be very therapeutic. When you do not know who to talk to, journal. Sit in the quiet, put your guard down, and let the pen move, expressing every thought and feeling of your heart. Also try starting a gratitude page, which will help you see the blessings and light during the dark times.

Find Community: Infertility is an incredibly isolating cross, especially in Catholic circles as you try to find your place as the couple with no kids, or perhaps one or two, when all your friends are expecting number five. Know that you are not alone. There are so many other women who are suffering in silence.

Find a group on social media. Have coffee dates with other women who are going through similar experiences. Start a group in your church. You will be amazed at how many women will come forward. When pain strikes, it is easy to isolate ourselves even more because we think no one will understand. Resist the isolation and find community. Remember also that with a miscarriage or stillbirth, you do not have to tell everyone, because not every person will understand your pain. At the same time, do not feel like you can't tell *anyone.*

Grow in Your Marriage: Cling to your spouse. The statistics of marriage ending in divorce due to infertility and miscarriage are frightening. Studies show that couples who experience infertility are three times more likely to divorce, and those who suffer a miscarriage are 22 percent more likely.

Men and women grieve differently, often leaving the other spouse feeling isolated. Use this time as an opportunity to draw nearer to your spouse. Make a concerted effort to talk through the emotions, coming to a deeper understanding of where each of you are and what your needs are in finding healing. When it may seem easier to retreat from your spouse, make an effort to spend time with him or her. Enjoy having more movie nights, dinners out, quiet nights in, or weekends away.

Grow in Affection: If you have children on earth, draw closer to them by cuddling and hugging them more frequently. They might see your tears during your grieving, and that is okay. But never forget your blessings.

Avoid Triggers: Struggling to feel truly excited as another friend announces she is pregnant or feeling a pit in your stomach as you scroll through social media and see yet another ultrasound picture are not reasons to feel guilty. Allow yourself time and know what you can emotionally handle. Give yourself permission to avoid triggers, such as baby showers or seeing a pregnant friend or a friend who has a baby, until you are ready. Avoiding these situations does not make you weak, but will aid in the healing process.

Seek Medical Help: After a miscarriage, stillbirth, or infant loss, it is wise to schedule an appointment with your gynecologist. It is important to follow up on blood work, which sometimes can suggest some deficiencies and the need for medicine. When you feel you are ready, there may be instances where seeking out more medical care is needed. Physicians trained in NaProTechnology can help navigate and guide you through fertility care and hormone support therapy, and perhaps assist in finding answers to help heal your body. NaProTechnology (www.naprotechnology.com, www.fertilitycare.org) was founded by a devout Catholic, Dr. Thomas Hilgers, and the care given is completely in line with Catholic teaching, as it respects the procreative process as a gift between a husband and wife while aiding in support of the woman's natural abilities to conceive and carry a child.

Physical and Mental Health: Although it may seem like you will never feel like yourself again and you wonder when "normalcy" will set in, it is important to take care of your physical and mental health. That may mean seeking a counselor to help you talk through the grief or perhaps taking extended leave from work. Seeking out and engaging in activities that will lower your stress will also naturally help you feel peace. Going for nature walks might help ease your pain by taking your mind off your struggles. Surrounded by God's outdoor cathedral, we begin to breathe a little easier and realize that we have basic needs in life and one of them is to just breathe. Physical exercise combined with uplifting music can also help release tension. It might be helpful to pick up a new hobby, such as learning to watercolor or play a musical instrument, to help cope with your grief in a calm manner. Above all, be patient and gentle with yourself, as God is carrying you at this most trying moment of your life.

CHAPTER 19

For Those Who Support and Console the Grieving Heart

One of the seven Spiritual Works of Mercy is to comfort the sorrowful. For some reason, though, we forget this with those who lose a child due to miscarriage or stillbirth, possibly because it is so hidden or because we simply do not know how to respond. In many miscarriages, especially those in the first trimester, there seldom is an intact body, only the dream of a baby who would someday be held. Just because we did not get to hold a living child or even see an ultrasound does not mean that we ought to grieve any less than a mother who lost a child later in life. In fact, a miscarriage is so painful because in most cases we experienced the immense joy of finding out we were pregnant. Perhaps we even told a few close family members and friends. We started to pray about names we might choose and may even have purchased some baby clothes. Then, when our child died, our world crumbled in a matter of seconds. Meanwhile, some relatives, friends, and coworkers, especially those who have never lost a child, act as if nothing happened when they hear of our loss.

In the next few paragraphs, we are going to show how you can be like the Good Samaritan in the Gospel rather than the priest or Levite who "passed by on the other side" (Luke 10:32). To heal from a miscarriage, stillbirth, or infant loss, it is essential to the grieving heart to have people in their inner circle or even the random acquaintance to show compassion by binding up their wounds with oil and wine like the Good Samaritan. The following are practical ways to support someone who has lost a child — that is, to comfort the sorrowful.

Pray: Praying for the living and the dead is another one of the Spiritual Works of Mercy. We must pray that God will give the mother and father the strength to rediscover their peace and joy. We must pray daily for their healing of mind, body, and soul. Offering our Mass and Rosary intentions can be very powerful. In many cases, a miscarriage, stillbirth, or infant loss can be brought upon by some medical condition. We must pray that the doctors and counselors can assist our relative or friend. We should pray to the Holy Spirit to guide us to better serve their grieving heart. We must never cease to pray for our relatives or friends, even months or years later, especially when there are additional miscarriages.

Action: The Good Samaritan did not pray that someone would help the beaten-up man; instead, he assisted him. We can pour oil and wine on the grieving heart's wounds by sending a card or flowers, or by bringing a meal. Give the person a memorial gift, such as a Christmas ornament, a picture of Jesus or Mary with children, or an angel statue that will help them remember their child. Even the smallest gesture can bring great comfort when it seems no one else notices, acknowledges, or seems to care. Organize a special Mass in your parish or diocese for people who have lost a child. It is important to remember the father, too. Many people will ask the father, "How is your wife doing?" They forget that he also is suffering. The son he longed to play catch with or daughter he longed to tuck into bed is no more.

Words: While words may be the hardest thing to find or know how to formulate, the grieving heart longs to hear the words, "I am sorry for your loss," or "We are suffering with you." A hug and shared tears can go a long way. Even months, sometimes a year, after losing a child, we need to be asked, "How are you doing?" "How are you handling the miscarriage [or stillbirth or infant loss]?" or "Is there anything I can do to help you?" We cannot assume that our friend or relative is better just because time has passed. When you do not acknowledge the lost child or even the parents' pain, you are failing to show compassion. Silence can translate to a lack of empathy. You are passing on the other side of the road like the priest and Levite in the parable of the Good Samaritan. While it might be awkward or even painful to bring up the lost child, it is more painful to remain silent. We need to be like Our Lord, who is the Good Samaritan, by showing mercy and compassion to our wounded brothers and sisters. Some people may not like to talk about their deceased child or share their feelings, but by asking and offering a few simple words, you have shown that you care.

Space and Prudence: Understand that a grieving parent might be distant for a while because their heart needs some time with their spouse to process their tragic loss. Instead of taking it personally, use it as a time to respect their privacy and to let them know you are here for them should they want to talk on the phone or meet in person. If you get pregnant, especially around the time they lost their child, it is prudent not to share your good news immediately. Consider telling them in private or writing them a letter. You should not feel guilty that your child lived and theirs did not, but you should be mindful that they might not come to your baby's shower or Baptism — and do not take it personally. It is also prudent to avoid sending or talking about anything baby-related. While you want them to rejoice in your happiness, it is best you share this with other people, who have not lost a child recently. When your child is born, do not be afraid to ask the mother and father to hold them if you feel comfortable. Just because they lost a child does not mean they will have ill will toward your child or not want to hold the baby. In fact, they long to hold a child in their arms, for theirs have felt empty for so long.

Remember: Mark on your calendar the anniversary of your relative's or friend's child loss or due date and send them a text, card, or flowers on those dates. Often we feel sad when those nearest to us forget our birthday. How much more when we forget their sufferings when they needed us the most, and more important, forget the child they longed for?

CHAPTER 20

Ten Things Not to Say to People Who Have Lost a Child

1. You are still young; you can always have another one. Or: It is time to move on.
2. At least your child is in Heaven now.
3. Are you pregnant again? Or: Do you plan on trying again?
4. It just wasn't meant to be.
5. It was God's will. Or: This was God's plan.
6. There was probably something genetically wrong with your baby.
7. Buy a dog.
8. I know someone who went to Dr. [NAME] and had a successful pregnancy. Or: I heard of a way to prevent miscarriages.
9. I'm pregnant! *(Wait to share this news with someone who has recently lost a child.)*
10. Do you want to come to my baby shower next week [or month]?

Part IV

REFLECTIONS, PRAYERS, AND SCRIPTURE PASSAGES

CHAPTER 21

Reflections

Reflection from Mother Angelica

My Lord, the baby is dead!

Why, my Lord — dare I ask why? It will not hear the whisper of the wind or see the beauty of its parents' face — it will not see the beauty of Your creation or the flame of a sunrise. Why, my Lord?

"Why, my child — do you ask 'why'? Well, I will tell you why.

"You see, the child lives. Instead of the wind he hears the sound of angels singing before My throne. Instead of the beauty that passes he sees everlasting Beauty — he sees My face. He was created and lived a short time, so the image of his parents imprinted on his face may stand before Me as their personal intercessor. He knows secrets of Heaven unknown to men on earth. He laughs with a special joy that only the innocent possess. My ways are not the ways of man. I create for My Kingdom and each creature fills a place in that Kingdom that could not be filled by another. He was created for My joy and his parents' merits. He has never seen pain or sin. He has never felt hunger or pain. I breathed a soul into a seed, made it grow, and called it forth."

I am humbled before you, my Lord, for questioning Your wisdom, goodness, and love. I speak as a fool — forgive me. I acknowledge Your sovereign rights over life and death. I thank You for the life that began for so short a time to enjoy so long an Eternity.

A Letter from the Nursery of Heaven

Dear Mommy and Daddy,

It might be years, months, or just a few weeks since I dwelt in my little Heaven on earth, the tabernacle of my mother's womb. You might have even seen me on the ultrasound or heard my little rapid heartbeat. Even if you never did, I still felt your love. My little heart was beating for you because I knew you loved me. I couldn't wait for the day when you would hold me in your arms and call me by name, but that day never came.

Instead, our Heavenly Father called me to Himself, and He placed me in the most tender and loving arms, those of the Blessed Mother. Someday you will hold me and I cannot wait. For you that day might seem like an eternity, but for me, eternity is only a moment. Our Heavenly Father has prepared a place for you. If only you could see how beautiful Heaven is and how happy I am, your tears would be turned to joy. If only you knew how much God loves you and if only you could see His face and His Mother's, you would die of joy.

I pray for you every day and I will never cease praying for you until you are safe in our Father's House. Only a thin veil separates us. I know you miss me and I miss you both more than you know. Never forget that our separation is only temporary. Jesus told me He is with you always, even when those around you have forgotten your pain, even when you feel abandoned by Him. He is helping you carry your cross. Let Him help you. Let Him carry you. He too missed His Mother when He died on the Cross and left this world. He longed for the day when they would be reunited in Heaven. He longed for His mother's love and caresses.

Sometimes you wonder why God took me, meanwhile other family members and friends have never known such loss, one of the greatest sorrows of your life. You might ask why their children lived and why I didn't. When you get to Heaven, the Father will make known everything. His ways are not our ways. He only wants the best for you. Trust Him. For now, please know this, Mommy and Daddy — I am never far away. My cells live in you, Mommy, so a part of me will always be with you in a mysterious way. Talk to me and ask me to pray for you. I am before the throne of God. Name me if you haven't already. I am a person, fully alive. Thank you for cooperating with God to give me life. Even though my mission on earth was short, my mission in Heaven is only beginning.

Soon we will be together forever in Heaven where there will be no more tears, no more crosses, and no more distance. And I cannot wait for that day when I will hug you and never let you go. I am your child now and forever, but we are God's beloved children first. Do not fear, my dear parents. I am waiting for you in the Nursery of Heaven. When it is your time to come to Heaven, Jesus will take me from His Mother's arms and we will welcome you with the greatest love you have ever experienced. Goodbye, my beautiful parents. See you in a moment.

With all my love and hugs and kisses,
Your beloved child

A Treasured and Entrusted Child

Funeral Homily for Adelaide Marie Borofka
St. Paul's Church, April 26, 2021
Fr. Victor Feltes

The dominant culture in the days of Jesus' public ministry oftentimes did not treasure children. A firstborn baby boy might have value to a Roman father, but a baby who was a girl, or malformed, or disabled, or simply unwanted might be killed or abandoned in the woods, exposed to die. The early Christians, however, rejected infanticide and adopted foundlings, raising them as their own. This is reflected by a first-century Christian text called The Didache (also known as "The Lord's Teaching through the Twelve Apostles to the Nations") which commands: "You shall not procure an abortion, nor destroy a newborn child." From where did the Christians get this countercultural concern for all children, born and unborn? From our Lord Jesus Christ, of course.

Though children are small and weak, Jesus says, "See that you do not despise one of these little ones, for I say to you that their angels in heaven always look upon the face of my heavenly Father." They have no wealth or worldly power, but Jesus says, "Unless you turn and become like children, you will not enter the kingdom of heaven." Jesus, calling a child over and putting His arms around him, says, "Whoever humbles himself like this child is the greatest in the kingdom of heaven." Jesus says that children are to be treasured and loved like himself: "Whoever receives one child such as this in my name receives me." Jesus says, "Let the children come to me, and do not prevent them; for the kingdom of heaven belongs to such as these." In just the same way as a good shepherd hates to lose even one of his many sheep, Jesus says, "It is not the will of your heavenly Father that one of these little ones be lost." Indeed, "Jesus loves the little children, all the little children of the world."

So even when a child dies without Baptism, we can entrust them to God's mercy with great hope, that the love of God which has brought us into being will transform the painful mysteries of the Cross into a reunion of Easter joy. In the midst of any tragedy, we always have a general Christian hope that God will bring good out of what is bad. But in regards to little Adelaide it appears that God has granted us a special, particular consolation. This is Veronica's story, which she has given me permission to tell you, and which she wants me to share for your benefit.

On Easter Sunday, Veronica began to feel severe abdominal pain. She was admitted to Sacred Heart Hospital in Eau Claire with a blood pressure so high that she was in grave danger of suffering a stroke, even dying. Then, through an ultrasound, it was discovered that the child within her, the child she lovingly carried for seven months, no longer had a heartbeat. Around 2 a.m. on Monday, April 5, while she was in great physical and emotional pain, her husband, Zach, and their gathered family members were praying a Rosary with her. Veronica was praying along with them, off and on, as she could manage. And in the midst of all this painful suffering, as she paused with her eyes closed, she saw something. Even though Veronica is certain that she was awake at that moment, she beheld something remarkable. Before I describe Veronica's experience and what she saw, I will speak briefly about private revelation.

As Catholics we believe that Jesus is not dead, but risen and living. We believe that his saints in Heaven are all alive with him. We believe that Jesus and his saints and angels know us, that they care about us, and that they continue to lovingly help us here on earth. We believe visions, messages, and miracles still happen in our day. And sometimes instances of these phenomena are judged by the Church's authority to be "worthy of belief." However, unlike public revelation (which consists of Sacred Scripture and the apostolic teachings in the Deposit of Faith), private revelation, even when officially recognized by the Church, is not binding to be believed by all the faithful. I am not personally qualified to make any official judgment for the Church about private revelations, but I tell you: if I did not personally believe that what Veronica saw was of a heavenly origin, I would not be about to share it with you.

Veronica, with her eyes closed during that Rosary in the hospital, saw a woman standing before her bed. There were pretty, puffy, white clouds behind the woman and to each side of her. And rays of sunlight from the left peeked through gaps in the clouds. The woman wore a dazzling, bright white gown. The fabric of her beautiful, full-length dress looked like satin. It had a modest scoop neckline and sleeves that went down to her wrists. The woman also wore a blue, cathedral-length veil of traditional lace, which extended down to the floor. She was dressed similarly to a statue of the Blessed Virgin Mary from Germany which Veronica's grandfather had given her years before — a statue Veronica used to play with as a girl.

The woman had long, curly, dark hair, snow-white skin, and beautiful blue eyes which gazed at Veronica. The expression on the woman's face was very pleasant, calming, and peaceful, concerned for Veronica and reassuring. Veronica says, "She looked absolutely beautiful and gorgeous," such that "no model could compare." The woman's lips moved as she slowly spoke with a very feminine, light and calming, beautiful voice, which echoed with some reverberation. And this is what she said: "Veronica, do not be afraid. I will take care of this child as I have taken care of my Son, Jesus. Do not worry and do not cry."

In this vision, Veronica held in her hands her swaddled baby, wrapped in the gray swaddling cloth she had bought for its birth. (Veronica did not yet know whether she had a girl or a boy, since Adelaide had not yet been delivered.) Hearing the Virgin Mary's words gave her great relief for, Veronica reflected, who could be better than the Blessed Mother to care for her lost child? Veronica raised up her arms in the vision, completely entrusting her child to Mary. Mysteriously, Mary remained where she stood but seemed to come closer. Veronica says, "I handed her my child and then she was gone." The entire vision was very brief, perhaps just ten or fifteen seconds, about the length of one Hail Mary prayer.

Veronica was left with feelings of peace, calm, reassurance that everything was okay — and wonder that the Blessed Mother would make herself known to her. Veronica did not share her story right away — she was worried people might think she was crazy — but after this vision she began comforting those gathered around her bedside. When her mother began to cry, Veronica told her, "Don't cry, you don't have to cry." As St. Paul told the Corinthians, "[God] encourages us in our every affliction, so that we may be able to encourage those who are in any affliction with the encouragement with which we ourselves are comforted by God."

Veronica is saddened, of course, still grieving and mourning, but not crushed or depressed like one might expect. She always had faith in God and Jesus Christ, but this experience has reinforced it, and she desires the same growth in Christian faith for you. "There's beauty in the suffering," she told me, adding, "I just want everyone to know what I know and to feel the peace that I feel with God and His love." This is the Lord Jesus Christ's wish for you, too. Clouds may limit our vision in this world, preventing us from seeing all that God is up to, but even in the hardest times rays of light still shine through. This light comes from the Lord Jesus who loves us, who treasures little Adelaide, and who also treasures you.

CHAPTER 22

Prayers

Blessing of Parents after a Miscarriage or Stillbirth

In times of death and grief the Christian turns to the Lord for consolation and strength. This is especially true when a child dies before birth. This blessing is to be used by a layperson and is provided to assist the parents in their grief and console them with the blessing of God.

Introductory Rites

All make the Sign of the Cross. The leader begins:

Let us praise the Father of mercies,
the God of all consolation.
Blessed be God forever.
℟. *Blessed be God forever.*

In the following or similar words, the leader prepares those present for the blessing.

For those who trust in God,
in the pain of sorrow there is consolation,
in the face of despair there is hope,
in the midst of death there is life.

N. and N., as we mourn the death of your child,
we place ourselves in the hands of God
and ask for strength, for healing, and for love.

Reading of the Word of God

One of those present or the leader reads a text of Sacred Scripture (Lam. 3:17–26).

Listen to the words of the book of Lamentations:

My soul is deprived of peace,
I have forgotten what happiness is;
I tell myself my future is lost,
all that I hope for from the Lord.

The thought of my homeless poverty
is wormwood and gall;
Remembering it over and over,
leaves my soul downcast within me.

But I will call this to mind,
as my reason to have hope:
The favors of the Lord are not exhausted,
his mercies are not spent;
They are renewed each morning,
so great is his faithfulness.
My portion is the Lord, says my soul;
therefore I will hope in him.

Good is the Lord to one who waits for him,
to the soul that seeks him;
It is good to hope in silence for the saving help of the Lord.

The word of the Lord.
℟. *Thanks be to God.*

Or: Isaiah 49:8–13 — In a time of favor I answer you, on the day of salvation I help you.
Romans 8:18–27 — In hope we were saved.
Romans 8:26–31 — If God is for us, who can be against us?
Colossians 1:9–12 — We have been praying for you unceasingly.
Hebrews 5:7–10 — Christ intercedes for us.
Luke 22:39–46 — Agony in the garden.

As circumstances suggest, one of the following responsorial psalms may be sung, or some other suitable song.

℟. To you, O Lord, I lift up my soul.

Psalm 25

Your ways, O LORD, make known to me; / teach me your paths, / Guide me in your truth and teach me, / for you are God my savior,/ and for you I wait all the day. ℟.

Remember that your compassion, O LORD, / and your kindness are from of old. / The sins of my youth and my frailties remember not; / in your kindness remember me/ because of your goodness, O LORD. ℟.

Look toward me, and have pity on me, / for I am alone and afflicted. / Relieve the troubles of my heart, / and bring me out of my distress. ℟.

Preserve my life, and rescue me; / let me not be put to shame, for I take refuge in you. / Let integrity and uprightness preserve me, / because I wait for you, O LORD. ℟.

Psalm 143:1, 5–6, 8, 10 ℟. *(v. 1) O Lord, hear my prayer.*

Intercessions

The intercessions are then said.

Let us pray to God, who throughout the ages
has heard the cries of parents.

℟. *Lord, hear our prayer.*

For N. and N., who know the pain of grief, that they may be comforted,
we pray to the Lord. ℟.

For this family, that it may find new hope in the midst of suffering,
we pray to the Lord. ℟.

For these parents, that they may learn from the example of Mary, who grieved by the cross of her Son,
we pray to the Lord. ℟.

For all who have suffered the loss of a child, that Christ may be their support,
we pray to the Lord. ℟.

After the intercessions, the leader invites all present to say the Lord's Prayer.

Prayer of Blessing

The leader says the prayer of blessing with hands joined.

Compassionate God,
soothe the hearts of N. and N.,
and grant that through the prayers of Mary,
who grieved by the Cross of her Son,
you may enlighten their faith,
give hope to their hearts,
and peace to their lives.

Lord, grant mercy to all the members of this family
and comfort them with the hope
that one day we will all live with You,
with Your Son Jesus Christ, and the Holy Spirit,
forever and ever.
℟. *Amen.*

Or:

Lord, God of all creation,
we bless and thank You for Your tender care.
Receive this life You created in love
and comfort Your faithful people in their time of loss
with the assurance of Your unfailing mercy.
Through Christ Our Lord.
℟. *Amen.*

Concluding Rite

The leader concludes the rite by signing himself or herself with the Sign of the Cross and saying:

May God give us peace in our sorrow,
consolation in our grief,
and strength to accept His will in all things
℟. *Amen.*

Order for the Naming and Commendation of an Infant Who Died before Birth

Archdiocese of St. Louis, 2013

Introduction

1. It often happens among the people of God that a child dies prior to their birth due to miscarriage, an accident, or for some other reason. If an infant is alive, he/she should be baptized if this is possible (CIC, Can.871). However, when the baby is dead, baptism is not administered, since the sacraments of the Church are for the living.
2. In times of death and grief the Christian turns to the Lord for consolation and strength. In the *Order of Christian Funerals* the Church provides liturgical resources to assist the parents and other family members with their grief and help them deepen their faith and trust in the Lord. Accordingly, the *Order of Christian Funerals* contains adapted forms of the Vigil, the Funeral Liturgy and the Rite of Committal, which can be used for both baptized and unbaptized children and infants. In addition, a brief Rite of Final Commendation for an Infant is provided for use in the hospital, funeral home, or at the cemetery when the body is present.

The *Book of Blessings* contains an *Order for the Blessing of Parents after a Miscarriage* which is also found in a simplified form in *Catholic Household Blessings and Prayers.* This rite is intended to assist the parents in their grief and console them with the blessing of God. It may be used by a priest or a deacon, and also by a lay person, who follows the rite and prayers designated for a lay minister.

These rites are the primary liturgical sources which the minister will use in the pastoral care of the parents and family of an infant who has died before birth.

3. However, these rites and prayers do not always respond to the need of many parents to name their child and commend it in faith to the loving mercy of God, when it is not possible to celebrate the funeral liturgy or the rite of committal. The following rite is provided for use as a means of responding to these parental needs.

4. The Order for the Naming and Commendation of an Infant Who Died before Birth seeks to set the death of an infant within the context of faith, and to unite the grieving parents and family members to the merciful God, whose love was revealed to us in the death and resurrection of Jesus Christ. The rite is not intended to offer certainty to the parents, but to provide them with a celebration based on Christian faith and hope.

5. This rite is primarily used when the baptism of an infant is neither possible or permitted (see no. 1 above), and when it is not possible or desirable to celebrate the funeral liturgy or rite of committal. It may be used in addition to or in place of the rites mentioned in no. 2, above.

Nos. 13, 19, and 20 may be used by a minister who is called to baptize an infant, but finds the infant is already dead and no members of the family are present.

6. If the body of the infant is not present during the service, some other reminder of the child may be present during the celebration.

7. The term "minister" is used in this rite to refer to priests, deacons, or lay ministers. When a particular prayer is

reserved to a priest or deacon, the words "priest" or "deacon" are used. The rites and prayers proper to a lay person are so indicated in the rite.

Introductory Rites

8. When all have gathered, a suitable song may be sung.

   The minister says:

   In the name of the Father, and of the Son, and of the Holy Spirit.

   All make the sign of the cross and reply:

   Amen.

9. A minister who is a priest or deacon greets those present in the following or other suitable words, taken mainly from Sacred Scripture.

   May the peace and consolation of the Lord be with you.

   And all reply:

   And with your Spirit.

10. A lay minister greets those present in the following words:

    Let us praise the God of peace and consolation. Blessed be God forever.

    ℟. Blessed be God forever.

11. In the following or similar words, which should always be adapted to suit the particular situation, the minister prepares the parents and others present for the celebration.

    For those who trust in God,

    in the pain of sorrow there is consolation, in the face of despair there is hope, in the midst of death there is life.

    N. and N., as we mourn the death of your child we place ourselves in the hands of God and ask for strength, for healing and for love.

Naming of the Child

12. The minister then asks the parents to name their child.

    What name do you give your child?

    The parents respond: *N.*

13. If the body of the infant is present, the minister may then trace the sign of the cross on or over the body of the infant, and, if appropriate, may also invite the parents and others present to do the same. The minister first says:

    In the name of the Christian community I sign N. (or this child) with the sign of the cross [and I invite his/her parents (and those who are present) to do the same]

Reading of the Word of God

14. A reader, another person present, or the minister reads a text of Sacred Scripture.

Brothers and sisters, listen to the words of the Gospel of Mark: (Mark 10:13–16)

People were bringing children to Jesus that he might touch them, but the disciples rebuked the people. When Jesus saw this he became indignant and said to the disciples, "Let the children come to me; do not prevent them, for the kingdom of God belongs to such as these. Amen, I say to you, who ever does not accept the kingdom of God like a child will not enter it." Then he embraced the children and blessed them, placing his hands on them.

Or:

Isaiah 49:8–13

In a time of favor I answer you, on the day of salvation I help you.

Romans 8:18–27

In hope we were saved.

Romans 8:26–31

If God is for us, who can be against us?

Colossians 1:9–12

We have been praying for you unceasingly.

15. As circumstances suggest, the minister may give those present a brief explanation of the biblical text, so that they may understand through faith the meaning of the celebration.

16. If desired, the minister may bless the parents of the infant using the following blessing taken from the *Book of Blessing: Order for the Blessing of Parents after a Miscarriage.*

    The minister invites all to pray using these or similar words:

    Let us pray to God who throughout the ages has heard the cries of parents.

After a brief pause for silent prayer, a minister who is a priest or deacon says the prayer of blessing with hands outstretched over the parents; a lay minister says the prayer with hands joined.

Compassionate God,

console the hearts of N. and N.,

and grant that through the prayers of Mary,
who grieved by the cross of her Son,

you may enlighten their faith, give hope to their hearts,

and peace to their lives.

Lord, grant mercy to all the members of this family and comfort them with the hope that one day we will all live with you, with your Son Jesus Christ, and the Holy Spirit, forever and ever.

℟. Amen.

Lord, God of all creation, we bless and thank you for your tender care. Receive this life you created in love and comfort your people in their time of loss, with the assurance of your unfailing mercy. We ask this through Christ Our Lord.

℟. Amen.

Blessing of the Body

17. Using the following words, the minister blesses the body of the deceased child.

Trusting in Jesus, the loving Savior, who gathered children into his arms and blessed the little ones,

we now commend this infant [N.] to that same embrace of love, in the hope that he/she will rejoice and be happy in the presence of Christ.

Then all join the minister saying:

May the angels and saints lead him/her to the place of light and peace, where one day we will be brought together again.

The minister continues:

Lord Jesus,

lovingly receive this little child; bless him/her and take him/her to your Father. We ask this in hope, and we pray:

Lord, have mercy.

℟. Lord, have mercy.

Christ, have mercy.

℟. Christ, have mercy.

Lord, have mercy.

℟. Lord, have mercy.

The Lord's Prayer

18. Using the following or similar words, the minister invites those present to pray the Lord's Prayer.

    When Jesus gathered his disciples around him, he taught them to pray:

    All say:

    Our Father . . .

Prayer of Commendation

19. The minister then says the following prayer.

    Tender Shepherd of the flock,

    N. now lies cradled in your love. Soothe the hearts of his/her parents and bring peace to their lives.

    Enlighten their faith

    and give hope to their hearts.

    Loving God,

    grant mercy to your entire family in this time of suffering.

    Comfort us with the hope that this child [N]. lives with you and your Son, Jesus Christ, and the Holy Spirit,

    forever and ever.

    ℟. Amen.

Blessing

20. Using one of the following blessings, the minister blesses those present.

    a. A minister who is a priest or deacon says:

       May the God of all consolation bring you comfort and peace, in the name of the Father, + and of the Son, and of the Holy Spirit.

       ℟. Amen.

    b. A lay minister invokes God's blessing and signs himself or herself with the sign of the cross, saying:

       May the God of all consolation bring us comfort and peace,

       in the name of the Father, and of the Son, and of the Holy Spirit.

       ℟. Amen.

The celebration may end with a suitable song.

Novena to St. Ann and St. Joachim

St. Ann and St. Joachim,
grandparents of Jesus and parents of Mary,
we seek your intercession.
We beg you to direct all our actions
to the greater glory of God
and the salvation of souls.
Strengthen us when we are tempted,
console us during our trials,
help us when we are in need,
be with us in life and in death.

O Divine Savior,
we thank You for having chosen St. Ann and St. Joachim
to be the parents of our Blessed Mother Mary
and so to be your beloved grandparents.
We place ourselves under their patronage this day.
We recommend to them our families,
our children, and our grandchildren.
Keep them from all spiritual and physical harm.
Grant that they may ever grow
in greater love of God and others.

St. Ann and St. Joachim
we have many great needs.
We beg you to intercede for us
before the throne of your Divine Grandson.
All of us here have our special intentions,
our own special needs,
and we pray that through your intercession
our prayers may be granted. Amen.

[Mention your intention(s) here.]

Our Father ... Hail Mary ... Glory Be to the Father ...

St. Ann and St. Joachim, pray for us.

Novena to St. Louis and St. Zélie Martin

Patrick O'Hearn

Heavenly Father,

We praise and thank you for the gift of our lives. Most of all, we thank you for giving us the Holy Eucharist and the Holy Spirit, your two greatest gifts.

We thank you for your holy servants, St. Louis and St. Zélie Martin. They sanctified marriage by responding generously and heroically to your holy will through a life of virtue, surrender, and suffering. We ask through their intercession to hear our prayers for [*mention your requests here*].

Dear St. Louis and St. Zélie Martin, you who shed copious tears over the loss of your four children, please bring our humble petitions before the throne of God and Our Lady to turn their eyes of mercy toward us. Increase our confidence in God's goodness and help us to surrender with serenity to His holy will as you did on earth, especially when our sufferings seem unbearable. Amen.

Our Father … Hail Mary … Glory Be to the Father …

St. Louis and St. Zélie Martin, pray for us.

Prayer to the Sacred Heart of Jesus

Cassie Everts

Oh Jesus, I turn to your most loving Sacred Heart in this time of sorrow and grief. Bring comfort to my heart. In the complete brokenness I feel, fill me entirely with your love. When there are no words to express my anguish, give me a song to sing, so that I may still praise you even in the storm. Strengthen my spirit, so that I can endure the heaviness of this cross and unite it to yours, carrying it for your glory. In my confusion and anger, pour your mercy upon me so that I may always trust in your divine plan for my life. May I never lose hope, knowing that my baby is now with you in Heaven, allow my heart to rest in yours, Jesus. Amen.

Prayer to Our Mother of Sorrows

Patrick O'Hearn

O Mother of Sorrows, you who once held your son and Our Lord in your blessed arms both at His birth and at His death, please look with mercy and compassion on our sufferings and grant us peace in our sorrows. Please kiss our departed child/children (*name them*) for us and keep them safe in your mantle until we meet again. Help us to unite our sufferings with Jesus and please grant us healing, hope, and perseverance that we might join you forever in Heaven along with all our family members, friends, and those in most need of thy mercy. Amen.

A Prayer to St. Catherine of Sweden for Healing and Consolation after Miscarriage

Dear St. Catherine, patron of those who have suffered a miscarriage, you know the dangers that await unborn infants.

Please intercede for me that I may receive healing from the loss I have suffered.

My soul has been deprived of peace and I have forgotten what true happiness is.

As I mourn the loss of my child, I place myself in the hands of God and ask for strength to accept His will in all things, for consolation in my grief, and for peace in my sorrow.

Glorious St. Catherine, hear my prayers and ask that God, in good time, grant me a healthy baby who will become a true child of God. Amen.

A Prayer to St. Catherine of Sweden for a Healthy Pregnancy and for Avoiding Miscarriage

Dear St. Catherine, you know the temptations of mothers today as well as the dangers that await unborn infants.

Intercede for me that I may avoid miscarriage and bring forth a healthy baby who will become a true child of God.

Dear Heavenly Father, I thank and praise You for the gift of all human life.

I am most especially grateful for the new life within my womb — the unborn child forming deep within me.

Through the prayers of Mary, Mother of Jesus, and the intercession of St. Catherine of Sweden, I beg You to watch over and protect this little one inside my womb.

In Jesus' Name. Amen.

A Prayer to St. Catherine of Siena for Avoiding Miscarriage

Humble Virgin and Doctor of the Church,
in thirty-three years
you achieved great perfection
and became the counselor of popes.
You know the temptations of mothers today
as well as the dangers that await unborn infants.
Intercede for me
that I may avoid miscarriage
and bring forth a healthy baby
who will become a true child of God.
Also pray for all mothers,
that they may not resort to abortion
but help bring a new life into the world. Amen.

A Prayer to St. Gerard for Safe Delivery

O great St. Gerard, beloved servant of Jesus Christ, perfect imitator of your meek and humble Savior, and devoted child of the Mother of God, enkindle within my heart one spark of that heavenly fire of charity which glowed in your heart and made you an angel of love. O glorious St. Gerard, because when falsely accused of crime, you did bear, like your Divine Master, without murmur or complaint, the calumnies of wicked men, you have been raised up by God as the patron and protector of expectant mothers. Preserve me from danger and from the excessive pains accompanying childbirth, and shield the child which I now carry, that it may see the light of day and receive the purifying and life-giving waters of baptism through Jesus Christ Our Lord. Amen.

Litany of the Saints For those seeking to conceive and those who have lost a child

Patrick O'Hearn

Lord, have mercy on us. . . . . *Lord, have mercy on us.*
Christ, have mercy on us.. . . . .*Christ, have mercy on us.*
Lord, have mercy on us. . . . . *Lord, have mercy on us.*
Christ, hear us. . . . . *Christ, graciously hear us.*
God, the Father of Heaven, ... *have mercy on us.*
God the Son, Redeemer of the world, ... *have mercy on us.*
God the Holy Spirit, ... *have mercy on us.*
Holy Trinity, one God, ... *have mercy on us.*
Holy Mother of God, in whose womb
God was conceived, ... *pray for us.*
Our Mother of Sorrows, who lost Jesus
for three days and later on the Cross, ... *pray for us.*
Our Lady of Guadalupe, patroness of the unborn, ... *pray for us.*
St. Alphonsus Rodriguez, who lost three children, ... *pray for us.*
St. Ann, patron of childless women and
women in labor, ... *pray for us.*
Bl. Catalina de María Rodríguez, who lost
a stillborn daughter, ... *pray for us.*
St. Catherine of Siena, patron against miscarriages
and whose twin died at birth, ... *pray for us.*
St. Catherine of Sweden, patron against miscarriages, ... *pray for us.*
Servant of God Chiara Corbella Petrillo,
who lost two children, ... *pray for us.*
St. Collette, patron against infertility, ... *pray for us.*
Servants of God Cyprien and Daphrose Rugumba,
who lost seven children, ... *pray for us.*

St. Felicity of Carthage, who was martyred
while pregnant, ... *pray for us.*
St. Felicity of Rome, patron against the
death of children (seven sons martyred), ... *pray for us.*
Bl. Frédéric Ozanam, who lost multiple
children from miscarriage, ... *pray for us.*
St. Gerard, patron of childbirth and
pregnant women, ... *pray for us.*
St. Gianna, who miscarried two children,
patron of pregnant women and the unborn, ... *pray for us.*
St. Grellen, who brought a stillborn
baby back to life, ... *pray for us.*
Bl. Irmengard, patron against infertility and
for safety in multiple births, ... *pray for us.*
St. Joseph, patron of the Universal Church
and pregnant women, ... *pray for us.*
St. Josemaría Escrivá, who lost three
young siblings, ... *pray for us.*
St. Louis and St. Zélie Martin, who lost
four children and a stillborn nephew, ... *pray for us.*
St. Margaret of Antioch, patron of pregnant women,
and against milk loss for nursing, ... *pray for us.*
St. Rita of Cascia, patron against infertility
and for impossible causes, ... *pray for us.*
All you holy angels and Saints of God, ... *pray for us.*
Lamb of God, who takes away the
sins of the world, ... *Spare us, O Lord!*
Lamb of God, who takes away the
sins of the world, ... *Graciously hear us, O Lord!*
Lamb of God, who takes away the
sins of the world, ... *Have mercy on us.*

Christ, hear us. . . . . *Christ, graciously hear us.*

Lord Jesus, hear our prayer. . . . . *Lord Jesus, hear our prayer.*

Lord, have mercy on us. . . . . *Lord, have mercy on us.*

Christ, have mercy on us.. . . . .*Christ, have mercy on us.*

Lord, have mercy on us. . . . . *Lord, have mercy on us.*

CHAPTER 23

Scripture Passages

Isaiah 35:3–4 — Strengthen the weak hands,
and make firm the feeble knees.
Say to those who are of a fearful heart,
"Be strong, fear not!
Behold, your God
will come with vengeance,
with the recompense of God.
He will come and save you."

Isaiah 51:3 — For the Lord will comfort Zion;
he will comfort all her waste places,
and will make her wilderness like Eden,
her desert like the garden of the Lord;
joy and gladness will be found in her,
thanksgiving and the voice of song.

Psalm 55:22 — Cast your burden on
the Lord, and he will sustain you.

Psalm 113:9 — He gives the barren woman a home, making her the joyous mother of children. Praise the Lord!

Jeremiah 17:14 — Heal me, O Lord, and I shall be healed; save me, and I shall be saved; for thou art my praise.

Jeremiah 29:11 — For I know the plans I have for you, says the Lord, plans for welfare and not for evil, to give you a future and a hope.

Luke 1:37 — For with God nothing will be impossible.

Philippians 4:8 — Finally, brethren, whatever is true, whatever is honorable, whatever is just, whatever is pure, whatever is lovely, whatever is gracious, if there is any excellence, if there is anything worthy of praise, think about these things.

Revelation 21:4 — He will wipe away every tear from their eyes, and death shall be no more, neither shall there be mourning nor crying nor pain any more, for the former things have passed away.

Romans 15:13 — May the God of hope fill you with all joy and peace in believing, so that by the power of the Holy Spirit you may abound in hope.

Part V

TOOLS FOR THE JOURNEY

Contemplative Questions

Many of us have been told that we are not supposed to be angry with God. Why is it okay to be upset with God? How can I channel my anger toward God in a constructive way?

What steps will I take during the grieving process to help me find healing?

How will I get through the difficult days?

When triggers do arise, who can help me navigate through my feelings?

Many of us have been told to move on and that grieving is weakness. Why is it okay to grieve for our child, sometimes months or even years later? How can we grieve in a way that leads to healing and not despair?

We often think that the saints never dealt with depression and grief from losing a loved one. Yet the opposite is true. What lesson can we learn from the saints in their struggles?

We often feel like we must be self-reliant, especially when it comes to pain. Why is it a good thing to talk to a counselor or a priest, or to form a group?

What is the purpose of suffering? How can I see God's will in this suffering? Is there anything God is teaching me in my suffering?

Through our suffering, we often become more compassionate, which in Greek means "to suffer with." How can I become more compassionate to others through my own loss?

How can I remember my departed child? If I have children on earth, how can I draw nearer to them?

Additional Resources

Organizations

A Mom's Peace, a lay apostolate supporting mothers of miscarried and stillborn souls with burial, bereavement, and remembrance programs (www.amomspeace.org).

Catholic Miscarriage Support, a website that provides practical and spiritual support for Catholics who have lost a child to miscarriage (www.catholicmiscarriagesupport.com).

Elizabeth Ministry, supports families during the childbearing years and beyond with special care and support to those facing crisis and loss (www.elizabethministry.org).

Heaven's Gain Ministries, provides for the physical, emotional, and spiritual needs of families experiencing pregnancy loss — before, during, and after the delivery of their precious baby (www.heavensgain.org).

Held in Hope, a nonprofit that creates and distributes miscarriage boxes to equip and support women through their pregnancy loss (www.heldinhope.org).

Lily of the Valley, a Catholic apostolate that prayerfully serves families experiencing infertility, difficult prenatal diagnosis, postnatal medical challenges, and those who have had a pregnancy or infant loss (lotvministry.org).

Morgan's Place Cemetery, assists families through the grieving process by memory-making, birth planning, funeral and burial services, and post-partum support groups for parents (www.morgansplacecemetery.org).

Our Fruitful Love, a ministry from the Catholic Diocese of Arlington to give spiritual guidance, resources, and prayer for couples struggling with infertility, pregnancy loss, or stillbirth (www.ourfruitfullove.com).

Present in the Pain, a Catholic apostolate for mothers who have experienced the pain of child loss, especially through miscarriage, stillbirth, or infant loss (www.eileentully.com).

Red Bird Ministries, a nonprofit Catholic grief support ministry serving individuals and couples who have experienced child loss from pregnancy through adulthood (www.redbird.love).

Artwork

The Nursery of Heaven, a painting by Michael Corsini for the healing of those suffering from the loss of a child through miscarriage, stillbirth, or infant loss (www.michaelcorsini.com).

Blog

Lost Innocents Blog, offers practical help for miscarriage from an Orthodox Christian perspective. Provides specific details of what miscarrying a baby looks like (lostinnocentsblog.wordpress.com).

Books

The Grief of Dads: Support and Hope for Catholic Fathers Navigating Child Loss by Patrick O'Hearn and Bryan Feger with Kelly and Ryan Breaux (Ave Maria Press) — a book to help Catholic men experience healing after child loss.

Jellybean: A Baby's Journey to Heaven by Theoni Bell (Holy Heroes) — a children's picture book for families grieving after baby loss.

Our Lady of Sorrows: Devotion to Mary's Seven Sorrows for Children by Patrick O'Hearn (Sophia Institute Press) — a book to help children understand Mary's sufferings as well as their own.

Parents of the Saints: The Hidden Heroes behind Our Favorite Saints by Patrick O'Hearn (TAN Books) — a book that helps parents raise saints, but also reveals how to surrender to God in the midst of suffering, especially child loss.

Counseling

CatholicTherapists.com, an online resource that will help you find a Catholic therapist (www.catholictherapists.com).

Holistic Healing

Global Healing, offers a variety of natural remedies, such as a liver detox program, which helped Amanda O'Hearn conceive a child after six years of infertility (www.globalhealing.com).

Medical

Saint Paul VI Institute, the only medical institute of its kind that specializes in research, diagnosis, and treatment of procreative and women's healthcare within a pro-life ethic (www.popepaulvi.com).

Music

Beauty Unnoticed, the sound of a mother's broken heart being healed. Download the *Beauty Unnoticed* app or stream Danielle Rose's album wherever you listen (www.daniellerose.org).

Bibliography

American College of Obstetricians and Gynecologists. "Early Pregnancy Loss." Practice Bulletin no. 200. November 2018. https://www.acog.org/Clinical-Guidance-and-Publications/Practice-Bulletins/Committee-on-Practice-Bulletins-Gynecology/Early-Pregnancy-Loss.

American Pregnancy Association. "Symptoms and Signs of Miscarriage." Accessed April 26, 2024. https://americanpregnancy.org/getting-pregnant/pregnancy-loss/signs-of-miscarriage/.

Angelica, Mother M. "Miscarriage Prayer" (In Part 4, titled "Reflection from Mother Angelica"). EWTN. Accessed April 26, 2024. https://www.ewtn.com/catholicism/devotions/miscarriage-prayer-351.

"The Beatification of Frédéric Ozanam," The Holy See. https://www.vatican.va/jubilee_2000/magazine/documents/ju_mag_01091997_p-16_en.html.

Bennett, Caitrin. *Holier Matrimony: Rediscover the Church's Gifts to Married People.* Stockbridge, MA: Marian Press, 2024.

Centers for Disease Control and Prevention. "What Is Stillbirth?" Last reviewed September 29, 2022. https://www.cdc.gov/ncbddd/stillbirth/facts.html.

Centers for Disease Control and Prevention. "Pregnancy and Infant Loss." Last reviewed September 30, 2022. https://www.cdc.gov/ncbddd/stillbirth/features/pregnancy-infant-loss.html.

De Tarrazi, Amin A., and Fr. Ronald Ramson, eds. *Ozanam: Husband and Father, Champion of Truth and Justice, Lover of the Poor, Founder of the Society of St. Vincent de Paul.* Strasbourg, France: Éditions du Signe, 1997.

Ellis, Mark. "Mary Oversees Nursery in Heaven, Burpos Say." God Reports. May 6, 2014. https://www.godreports.com/2014/05/mother-mary-oversees-nursery-in-heaven-burpos-say/.

Hunter-Kilmer, Meg. "Saints Who Lost Children to Miscarriage." Aleteia. September 26, 2020. https://aleteia.org/2020/09/26/saints-who-lost-a-child-to-miscarriage/.

International Theological Commission. "The Hope of Salvation for Infants Who Die without Being Baptised." The Holy See. January 19, 2007. https://www.vatican.va/roman_curia/congregations/cfaith/cti_documents/rc_con_cfaith_doc_20070419_un-baptised-infants_en.html.

The Journey of Our Love: The Letters of Saint Gianna Beretta and Pietro Molla. Edited by Elio Guerriero. Boston: Pauline Books & Media, 2014.

Martin, St. Zélie, and St. Louis Martin. *A Call to a Deeper Love.* Edited by Frances Renda. Translated by Ann Connors Hess. Staten Island, NY: St. Paul's, 2011.

Molla, Pietro, and Elio Guerriero. *Saint Gianna Molla: Wife, Mother, Doctor.* Translated by James G. Colbert. San Francisco: Ignatius Press, 2004.

"Novena to St. Anne and St. Joachim." Ascension Press. Accessed April 26, 2024. https://ascensionpress.com/pages/novena-to-st-anne-and-st-joachim.

O'Hearn, Patrick. *Courtship of the Saints: How the Saints Met Their Spouses.* Gastonia, NC: TAN Books, 2023.

Pelucchi, Giuliana. *St. Gianna, Her Life of Joy and Heroic Sacrifice.* Boston: Pauline Books & Media, 2019.

"Prayer to Avoid a Miscarriage (To St. Catherine of Siena)." Catholic Doors Ministry. Accessed April 26, 2024. http://www.catholicdoors.com/prayers/english5/p03125.htm.

"Prayer to St. Gerard for Safe Delivery." At Anna Rapp, *To Make a Catholic Mommy* (blog). October 22, 2023. https://www.tomakeamommy.com/st-gerard-majella-patron-saint-of-trying-to-conceive/.

Prayers to St. Catherine of Sweden. At Anna Rapp, *To Make a Catholic Mommy* (blog). October 1, 2023. https://www.tomakeamommy.com/praying-to-st-catherine-of-sweden-for-healing-and-protection-from-miscarriage.

"Quotes Frédéric Ozanam." Vincentian Formation Network. Accessed April 26, 2024. https://vincentians.com/en/quotes-collection/frederic-ozanam-quotes/.

Taylor, Barbara Brown. *Gospel Medicine.* Cambridge, MA: Cowley Publications, 1995.

"This Argentine Nun's Cause for Beatification Is Advancing." Catholic News Agency. January 25, 2017. https://www.catholicnewsagency.com/news/35294/this-argentine-nuns-cause-for-beatification-is-advancing.

Troisi, Simone, and Christiana Paccini. *Chiara Corbella Petrillo: A Witness to Joy.* Translated by Charlotte J. Fasi. Manchester, NH: Sophia Institute Press, 2015.

Vazquez de Prada, Andrés. *The Founder of Opus Dei: The Life of Josemaria Escrivá*. Vol. 1, *The Early Years*. Princeton, NJ: Scepter, 2001.

About the Authors

Cassie Everts is a wife, mother, author, and speaker. She is the mother to five little ones in Heaven and six children on earth. Her writing has appeared at Catholic Exchange and Blessed Is She. She is a former producer at Relevant Radio and blogs at EverydayAnn.com. Cassie holds degrees in theology and communication arts from Franciscan University.

Patrick O'Hearn is a husband and father of four children, two in Heaven. He has authored or coauthored seven books, including *Parents of the Saints, Courtship of the Saints, The Shepherd at the Crib and the Cross, The Grief of Dads* (coauthor), *Go and Fear Nothing,* and *Our Lady of Sorrows*. He holds a master's degree in education from Franciscan University. You can visit his website at patrickrohearn.com.

If you wish to receive bulk pricing or want to pay it forward by ordering several copies for various bereavement ministries, contact Sophia Institute Press:

customerservice@sophiainstitute.com

Sophia Institute

Sophia Institute is a nonprofit institution that seeks to nurture the spiritual, moral, and cultural life of souls and to spread the gospel of Christ in conformity with the authentic teachings of the Roman Catholic Church.

Sophia Institute Press fulfills this mission by offering translations, reprints, and new publications that afford readers a rich source of the enduring wisdom of mankind.

Sophia Institute also operates the popular online resource CatholicExchange.com. *Catholic Exchange* provides world news from a Catholic perspective as well as daily devotionals and articles that will help readers to grow in holiness and live a life consistent with the teachings of the Church.

In 2013, Sophia Institute launched Sophia Institute for Teachers to renew and rebuild Catholic culture through service to Catholic education. With the goal of nurturing the spiritual, moral, and cultural life of souls, and an abiding respect for the role and work of teachers, we strive to provide materials and programs that are at once enlightening to the mind and ennobling to the heart; faithful and complete, as well as useful and practical.

Sophia Institute gratefully recognizes the Solidarity Association for preserving and encouraging the growth of our apostolate over the course of many years. Without their generous and timely support, this book would not be in your hands.

www.SophiaInstitute.com
www.CatholicExchange.com
www.SophiaTeachers.org

Sophia Institute Press is a registered trademark of Sophia Institute.
Sophia Institute is a tax-exempt institution as defined by the
Internal Revenue Code, Section 501(c)(3). Tax ID 22-2548708.